Diagnostic Radiology in Clinical Medicine

Diagnostic Radiology in Clinical Medicine

SECOND EDITION

ROSALIND H. TROUPIN, M.D.
Associate Professor of Radiology
University of Pennsylvania
Philadelphia, Pennsylvania

Illustrations by
Phyllis Wood
and
Charlotte P. Kaiser

YEAR BOOK MEDICAL PUBLISHERS, INC.
Chicago • London

Reprinted, May 1980

Library of Congress Cataloging in Publication Data
Troupin, Rosalind H.
    Diagnostic radiology in clinical medicine.

    Bibliography: p.
    Includes index.
    1.   Diagnosis, Radioscopic.   I.   Title.
[DNLM: 1.   Radiography.   WN200 T861d]
RC78.T78   1978   616.07'572   78-52544
ISBN 0-8151-8851-X

FOREWORD

IT IS A PLEASURE to have an opportunity to express my admiration for this manual. The author has a clear understanding of the point of view of the medical student and spells out exactly the kind of information students need about radiology and radiologic procedures. The manual is admirably well written in clear, succinct language, displays continuously humane, compassionate concern for the welfare and comfort of the patient being studied and invokes common sense logic with regard to the choice of procedure and the preparation of the patient. Certainly this book will relieve instructors of the necessity of reiterating for group after group of students important information about the practice of radiology. I know of no other source in which students can find the answers to their questions presented in so practical and readable a way. This one is right up to date, moreover.

LUCY FRANK SQUIRE, M.D.
August, 1977

ACKNOWLEDGMENTS

THIS MANUAL had its origins in a series of handouts used with film-reading sessions for medical students. With each passing semester, students helped me find better ways to do these write-ups, and the incessant revisions were patiently typed and copied by Joanne Forehand. It may have been accidental that the handouts were one day stapled together as a "syllabus."

Students visiting the University of Washington suggested that the write-ups might fit into their home curricula. In 1973 Year Book Medical Publishers, Inc. enabled the syllabus to go "public." Because of the extraordinary developments in radiology as new technology and concepts have emerged during the last 5 years, revision of the manual is necessary. In addition, students have asked that radiographic images be used in the new edition (providing it wouldn't increase the cost).

Lucy Frank Squire studied the incoherent draft of the original manual in detail, tried it on some of her students and subsequently offered excellent suggestions and advice. Incredibly, she willingly did this again in 1977 with the new edition, once more providing a constructive critique.

I am indebted to my chairman, Mel Figley, for his support and encouragement throughout the project. Two medical illustrators, Phyllis Wood and, more recently, Charlotte Kaiser, have used their skill and imagination to transform complex radiographic images into deceptively simple line drawings to facilitate learning and retention. Photographers Bill Holmes, Pat Siedlak and Doug Jones did their part with expertise and enthusiasm and were delightful collaborators. Anne Brunke coped with the manuscript and its author efficiently and cheerfully as revisions kept appearing by her typewriter. She laundered my sloppy references, researched ambiguous x-ray cost lists and kept everything moving in the right direction. Later, Gwen Reece was of major help in the preparation of the second printing.

My radiologic colleagues in Seattle contributed their time and case material very generously. I am indebted to Gerold Garrett, Steve Carter, Jack Hirsch, Howard Ricketts, Charles Rohrmann, Laurence Cromwell, Sue Conrad, Warwick Harvey-Smith, Asher Nov, Jimmy Rogers, Max Wolf, Julie Engel and Nicole Bolender for their help.

I am very grateful to those people and to my husband, Allan, and children, Mark and Barbara, who seem to be surviving my preoccupations and labilities.

MESSAGE TO TEACHERS OF RADIOLOGY

An editorial by the author

CURRICULUM REORGANIZATION in many medical schools has required us to modify the format in which we teach diagnostic radiology. The early integration of basic and clinical sciences into a systems-oriented approach has invited illustrative radiologic anatomy and pathology into each of these units. In lectures, demonstrations and correlative conferences we expose students to a great deal of rather hasty film viewing, but if we do it effectively, they do come to recognize many common patterns and images. Only later, during formal instruction in clinical radiology, is there time to encourage students to analyze nonclassical images logically and to understand the practical integration of x-ray studies with patient care.

Another major curriculum change has been the creation of large blocks of elective time. As a result, enormous numbers of eager, highly motivated students are presenting themselves to radiology departments seeking full-time instruction and participation. Some are, or will become, interested in a career in radiology. The majority, however, basically plan on becoming good physicians and recognize that they need additional practical information. Providing them with this on a repetitive basis throughout the academic year is a real challenge to departments with multiple functions and finite resources.

Many respected radiologic educators are currently pursuing ways to present the basic core of information in attractive self-instructional modes. When this is accomplished, faculty contact time can be diverted to discussions of more complex situations and insights into new developments and alternatives. Texts, workbooks, tapes, slides and film packets are all making their contribution. Initially, there *should* be an inefficient overlap of effort in order to amass and evaluate a large volume of instructional material. An eventual goal, however, might be a process of selection, duplication and dissemination of portions of this material. Local modification and periodic revision are highly desirable, but ultimately a basic "core" of high quality self-instructional material could be universally available.

This manual is one attempt to answer questions we are asked dozens of times each week. I hope you find it helpful in teaching or that it encourages you to write a better one for all of us to use. I would be grateful for comments or suggestions from teachers and students, who can contact me at the Department of Radiology, Hospital of the University of Pennsylvania, in Philadelphia.

ROSALIND HILSEN TROUPIN

July 14, 1978

CONTENTS

1

INTRODUCTORY PERSPECTIVES

Radiology in Clinical Medicine

THAT X-RAY EXAMINATIONS have assumed an increasingly major role in the overall evaluation of the sick and the injured is shown both by the heavy utilization of "standard" studies and by an enormous proliferation of "special procedures." Initially this manual was designed as a guide to radiologic fact and philosophy for the University of Washington medical student as he began his first clinical responsibilities. It has become apparent, however, that student-clinicians in later courses and training positions continue to find the approach helpful.

The first time around, the manual is best used in conjunction with film interpretation tutorials. It should supplement readings in one of the attractively illustrated texts, such as Squire,[1] Meschan,[2] Sutton[3] or Paul and Juhl.[4] Most chapters of the manual begin with a how-to-look-at and what-to-look-for kind of summary that should be studied while a representative examination is viewed. Illustrative sketches are deliberately exaggerated to emphasize significant points in your mind and will always be more striking than the original radiographs. The written lists, summaries and "rules" are the distillate of a large body of material. Summaries describe what is true *most* of the time and obviously do not dwell on uncommon exceptions. As clinical circumstances develop, you are urged to pursue more definitive, comprehensive references.

During this introductory survey of radiology, you will obviously want to learn calm, effective methods of analyzing the common x-ray examinations. You will be pleased to find that a systematic technique of looking at each film, coupled with the

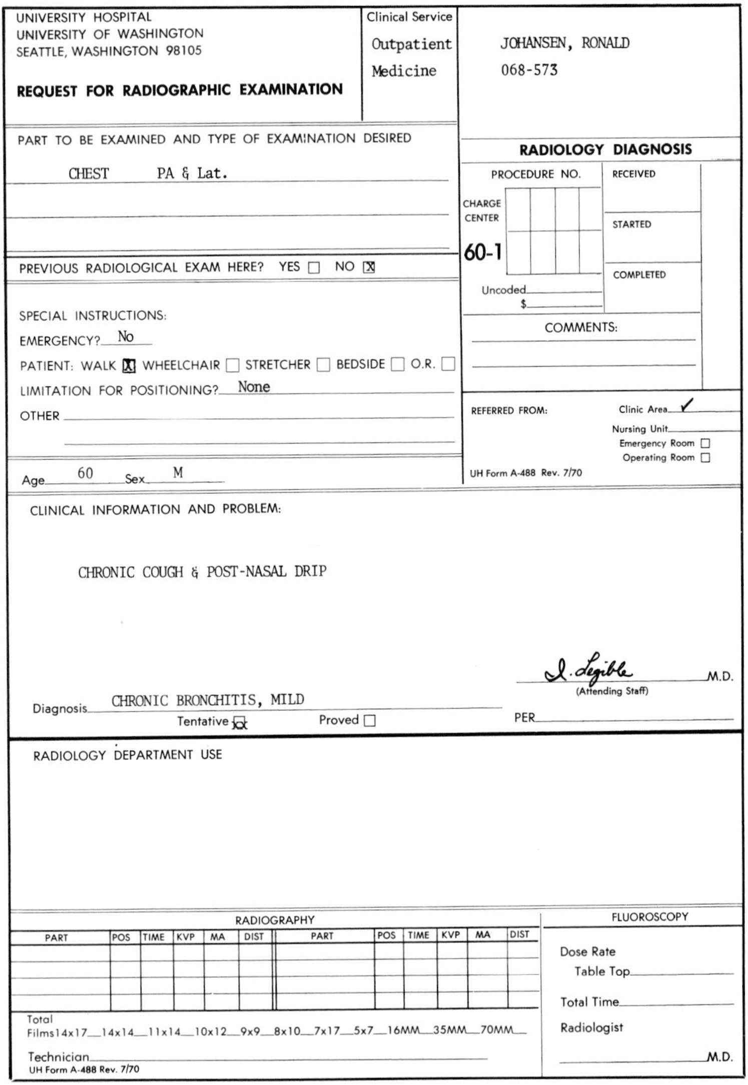

UNIVERSITY HOSPITAL UNIVERSITY OF WASHINGTON SEATTLE, WASHINGTON 98105	Clinical Service	JOHANSEN, RONALD
REQUEST FOR RADIOGRAPHIC EXAMINATION	Outpatient Medicine	068-573

PART TO BE EXAMINED AND TYPE OF EXAMINATION DESIRED

CHEST   PA & Lat.

RADIOLOGY DIAGNOSIS

PROCEDURE NO.	RECEIVED
CHARGE CENTER	STARTED
60-1	COMPLETED
Uncoded $	

PREVIOUS RADIOLOGICAL EXAM HERE?   YES ☐   NO ☒

COMMENTS:

SPECIAL INSTRUCTIONS:
EMERGENCY? No
PATIENT: WALK ☒ WHEELCHAIR ☐ STRETCHER ☐ BEDSIDE ☐ O.R. ☐
LIMITATION FOR POSITIONING? None
OTHER _____

REFERRED FROM: Clinic Area ✓
Nursing Unit _____
Emergency Room ☐
Operating Room ☐

Age 60   Sex M

UH Form A-488 Rev. 7/70

CLINICAL INFORMATION AND PROBLEM:

CHRONIC COUGH & POST-NASAL DRIP

I. Legible M.D.
(Attending Staff)

Diagnosis CHRONIC BRONCHITIS, MILD
Tentative ☒   Proved ☐

PER _____

RADIOLOGY DEPARTMENT USE

RADIOGRAPHY

PART	POS	TIME	KVP	MA	DIST	PART	POS	TIME	KVP	MA	DIST

FLUOROSCOPY

Dose Rate
Table Top _____

Total Time _____

Radiologist
_____ M.D.

Total
Films 14x17__ 14x14__ 11x14__ 10x12__ 9x9__ 8x10__ 7x17__ 5x7__ 16MM__ 35MM__ 70MM__

Technician _____
UH Form A-488 Rev. 7/70

Fig 1–1. — X-ray request form.

knowledge you already possess of normal anatomy and patho-physiology, will permit you to detect and understand many abnormal images. In radiologic diagnosis, just as in your clinical evaluation of someone's illness, there is no substitute for an unhurried critical appraisal of the information. "Shooting from the hip," to elicit startled admiration from bystanders, has no place in responsible patient care.

A second, but not secondary, goal should be to familiarize yourself with the wide variety of x-ray studies available for solving clinical problems and with the specific circumstances under which you might sensibly request them. Developing these judgments requires considering the indications, yields, costs and hazards of various diagnostic procedures. A radiologist, familiar with these factors, can help you select the appropriate examination and can then perform a study specifically tailored to answer your clinical question.

When circumstances of time and place prevent verbal consultation between clinician and radiologist on relatively straightforward problems, the communication becomes your request and the radiologist's written report. Figure 1–1 is a sample of one x-ray request form. Although yours is probably different in design, it is similar in purpose. The information you provide permits the radiologist to examine your patient safely and decisively. Clerical personnel do not know clinical details and are likely to submit data that fail to relate to the specific problem being investigated. *If you want the best possible examination for your patient, the responsibility for filling out the requisition is yours.*

In written reports to you, the radiologist analyzes the image, discusses the entities that could be responsible for it and summarizes by interpreting his objective findings in the light of what he knows of the clinical circumstances. In this final and crucial step, many possibilities are discarded, while one or more others are strengthened. If the radiologist believes that a supplementary examination will result in greater diagnostic specificity, he or she will recommend that you consider it. A clinician-radiologist dialogue should then determine whether that diagnostic specificity will benefit the patient or whether hot pursuit of the irrelevant is being proposed.

Diagnostic X-Ray Charges

Radiologic examinations are expensive, if not to the individual patient then to his insurance company or to the taxpayer. Somewhere, somebody in the system pays the bill. Thoughtful selection of examinations rather than broad-spectrum groping should obviously guide your actions, always following the reasoning of "what for," rather than "why not."

The following list shows some typical charges, combining technical and professional fees. Substantial variations certainly exist, and you should revise this list for your own time and place.

Chest	$ 36	Upper GI series	$105
Abdomen	35	Barium enema	110
Extremity	31–35	Excretory urogram (IVP)	91
Spine (C, T or L)	43	Oral cholecystogram	63
Skull	51	Ultrasound, abdomen	146
Mammogram	62	Computed tomography, abdomen	180
		Endoscopic retrograde cholangiography	600
		Percutaneous cholangiogram	255
Pulmonary arteriogram	648	Myelogram	273
Renal arteriogram	622	Carotid and vertebral arteriograms	500
Coronary arteriogram	1000	Computed tomography, brain	225

RADIONUCLIDE SCANS	
Lung	$147
Liver	147
Brain	152
Thyroid	53
Bone	176

Radiation Exposure in Diagnostic Radiology

You need a few background facts to guide you in shaping your philosophy of radiologic utilization, as well as to prepare you to answer your patients' questions. You will find that members of the public, while very curious about radiation exposure and protection, are often uninformed or have even been misinformed by the lay literature. At some point you will be asked, "But isn't that too much x-ray for me, doctor?" You must be prepared to answer that question to the patient's satisfaction and your own.

Within months of Roentgen's discovery of x-rays in 1895, x-ray laboratories opened and began to provide diagnostic services for local referring physicians. The initial applications were for skeletal trauma, but information and techniques began developing exponentially as other body systems were explored and the boundaries of normality and disease were established. X-ray examinations were immediately and enthusiastically welcomed into medicine; the frustrating centuries of not being able to look "inside" (without literally doing so) were over. Discovery of the antitumor and anti-inflammatory properties of radiation led to early therapeutic applications. The potent anticancer techniques of modern radiation therapy have their roots in those explorations.

Only in later years did the potential biologic hazards of high doses of ionizing radiation emerge and become defined. This recognition was delayed because of the long latent period of the effect; 15, 20 or 30 years might elapse between the exposures and the consequences. The combined efforts of epidemiologists and radiation biologists have been needed to unearth some of now-classic examples of radiation carcinogenesis:

- skin cancer in physicians who routinely used fluoroscopy during reduction of fractures

- bone tumors in radium watch dial painters

- thyroid cancer following thymic irradiation in infancy

- leukemia in patients who had recurrent spine irradiation for arthritis

- breast cancer in survivors of atomic bomb blast

Other exposures have not yet had clearly documented effects—for instance, the use of fluoroscopy in the fitting of children's shoes.

Diagnostic examinations obviously involve far smaller radiation exposure. Even though the somatic effects are generally not a significant consideration, we still worry about potential genetic effects. A major goal of modern radiologic technology is to minimize exposure dose in diagnostic examinations. Examples of such techniques include limitation of the size of the exposed field, use of more sensitive film and use of image intensification for electronic amplification of the fluoroscopic image. The precise radiation output of the equipment is periodically calibrated; machines and rooms are lead-shielded to standardized specifications, and personnel are regularly monitored for radiation exposure.

The physician who contemplates installing and using x-ray equipment in his office undertakes a grave responsibility. Antiquated equipment, carelessly monitored and maintained, is a leading source of unnecessary exposure for patients and personnel.

With the recognition that the figures given below represent gross oversimplifications of complex data, they are nonetheless offered to provide you with some sense of numerical perspective. Wide variations exist among installations; accept these figures as providing only a rough order of magnitude.

SOME "TYPICAL" EXPOSURE LEVELS

Total body lethal dose for man (LD/50)		400 rad
Cancer therapy: a small carefully defined volume of tissue is treated; dose is divided into small daily increments over several weeks		6,000 rad
Tolerance of normal organs (damage likely to occur above those levels)		
Kidney		2,400 rad
Lens		1,000 rad
Common diagnostic examinations:[5] dose to the structure being studied is usually insignificant; it *is* pertinent, however, to consider gonadal dosage	GONADAL DOSE in rad	
	Male	Female
Chest	0.0001	0.0003
Barium enema	0.140	1.060
GI series	0.015	0.330
Excretory urogram	0.042	0.420
Lumbar spine	0.040	0.500

Genetic Effects of Radiation on the Species

Ionization in germ cells increases the mutation rate, and, unfortunately, most mutations are unfavorable. An educated conjecture is that 30 rad to the gonads may double the rate of "spontaneous" mutations.

We cannot assume that genetic recovery occurs following irradiation, and the implications of regarding effects as *cumulative* are immense. Stated another way, genetic hazard cannot be considered in terms of one examination of one patient but should be regarded in the light of *all* of the exposures of that patient during his or her reproductive life, the exposure of the entire population and the exposure of succeeding generations.

Sensitivity of the Developing Fetus

It is well established that the developing embryo is extremely radiosensitive, especially during the earliest stages — from fertilization through organogenesis. In early mouse embryos, 15 rad can cause profound central nervous system anomalies; 5 rad can increase the intrauterine mortality by 10%.

It is critical to realize that at a comparable stage your patient may not yet know that she is pregnant.

You can avoid this potential hazard by scheduling nonemergency workups on women of childbearing age to correspond with menses or the week thereafter.

Although the risk of gross anomalies diminishes after organogenesis, the fetus remains very sensitive. Increasing data indicate that the risk of leukemia is substantially increased in children whose mothers had x-ray pelvimetry during pregnancy. It is the practice in some countries to recommend therapeutic abortion if the fetus has been exposed to 10 rad.

In the final analysis, responsible medical judgment must weigh the relative risks and potential benefits as each patient and each examination is contemplated. A procedure that furnishes an important diagnosis and leads to needed therapy should never be withheld. The unnecessary examination *is* "too much x-ray."

The Nature of the Radiographic Image

Generation of X-rays

The heated cathode filament in a vacuum tube "boils off" electrons, which are then accelerated across a very high voltage to strike a tungsten anode (Fig 1–2). X-rays, a form of electromagnetic energy, are emitted from this target. At the same time, heat is produced. The vacuum tube must be housed in a structure that provides cooling, shielding from electrical shock and absorption of all radiation other than the controlled beam. This emerging x-ray beam is then "coned down" to desired size and shape by lead shutters or collimators. Use of a higher kilovoltage generates x-rays with shorter wavelengths and greater penetrating power.

Differential Absorption in Tissue

The final image on the film results from differential absorption of the x-rays by the interposed body part. This absorption is dependent on both the volume and the density of the tissues being traversed (Fig 1–3).

A given thickness of bone will absorb more x-rays than will

Fig 1–2. – Clinical radiography.

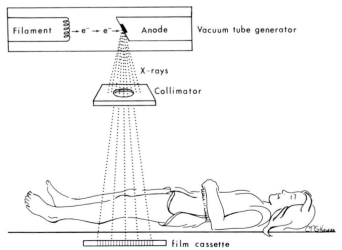

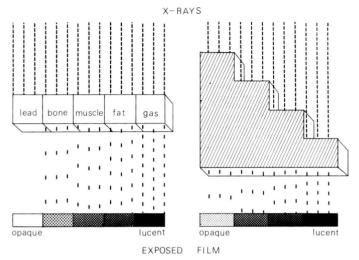

Fig 1–3. — X-ray absorption relates to density and volume of tissue traversed.

blood, muscle or liver; those tissues will absorb more than fat. Those are the differences that provide demarcation of anatomic planes and pathologic processes.

Film Exposure

X-ray film is composed of clear plastic base covered by an emulsion containing silver bromide. Light or x-rays cause a physicochemical alteration in the silver, which blackens when the film is developed in suitable chemicals. Blackening or exposure of the given area is an indicator of the amount of radiation which "got through" the object, i.e., there is not much blackening under a bone or under a great thickness of soft tissue. The term for this dense, white area on an x-ray film is *radiopacity*. A blackened area where x-ray absorption was less is called a *radiolucency*.

Geometric Effects

Variations in relative and absolute filming distances will produce striking alterations in image size (Fig 1–4). When

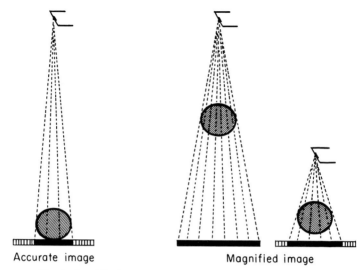

Accurate image   Magnified image

Fig 1–4. — Filming geometry and magnification effects.

that "image" is the outline of your patient's heart or kidneys the validity of comparing current and past measurements depends on whether the filming geometry has been duplicated.

2

CHEST FILMS

THE CHEST is an excellent place to begin development of your radiologic expertise. Its contents are revealingly displayed in an attractive variety of tissue densities packed closely together and providing natural contrasts. A chest x-ray is the one you will be requesting with greatest frequency and is the one you are most likely to find yourself viewing independently. It is unlikely that you will make a decision about an adrenal venogram without the aid of the radiologist or his report. You may, however, be the first person to see the chest film on your accident victim, and you will need to recognize the pneumothorax that requires your prompt action. Finally, chest filming is an area in which it is very easy to be misled into important errors by technical factors, and the sooner you cope with these variations the better.

For many, chest film interpretation is a fascinating intellectual exercise. It is complex enough to be challenging, yet pathoradiologic correlation is often so good that recognition of the classic and analysis of the atypical may provide immediate answers.

Obviously you will need to keep things in perspective. Your healthy young patient with an acutely febrile, sputum-producing illness and right basilar rales *has* pneumonia. You need to identify the organism and hit it hard with an antibiotic to which it is sensitive. The chest x-ray is of greatest use to warn you of a complication such as excavation, empyema or atelectasis and to document adequate response to therapy. On the other hand, in patients presenting with acute chest pain, chronic dyspnea, episodic hemoptysis or unexplained fever, the chest film could show *anything,* and you and your radiologist must be prepared to get it all sorted out.

11

Study Method

Getting Organized

Before diving in, decide *how* this examination was performed. This point will significantly influence what you see and what valid conclusions may be drawn from the image.

PATIENT SITUATION

- Upright or supine?
- PA or AP? PA is radiologic shorthand for "the x-ray beam traverses the body part from posterior to anterior. The patient's chest is against the film."
- Inspiration or expiration?
- Straight on or rotated?
- Moving?

RADIOGRAPHIC TECHNIQUE

- X-ray tube closer to patient than the standard 6-foot distance.
- Underexposed (too light) or overexposed (too dark)—we goofed and should re-do it.
- Processing artifacts.

Question: Under conditions of portable bedside filming of an acutely ill patient, which factors would contribute to a misleadingly broad cardiac image?*

Analyzing the Film

Carefully scrutinize each listed area, but do not just gaze; actively seek out specific things that you know can happen (Fig 2–1).

---

*AP projection with short tube-to-patient distance will cause geometric magnification. (If that slowed you down, recheck Figure 1–4.) Supine position, probably with suboptimal inspiratory effort, will result in high diaphragms and a transversely oriented heart.

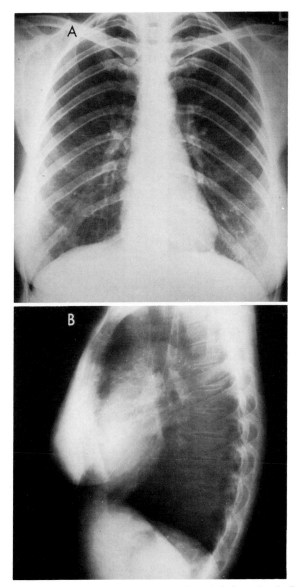

Fig 2–1.—Upright chest films of healthy adult female. **A,** PA view. **B,** lateral view.

Bones and Soft Tissues

Subcutaneous emphysema, fractures, rib notching, abnormal calcification, subdiaphragmatic air, splenomegaly, goiter. Be sure to include the neck, shoulders and upper abdomen in your search.

Mediastinum

Deviations or constrictions of the airway, dilatations or calcifications of the great vessels, mass lesions creating abnormal profiles, mediastinal shift.

Cardiac Image

Generalized or selective chamber enlargement, calcifications (more details later).

Pleura

Effusion, pneumothorax, thickening, calcification.

Hila

Adenopathy, masses, pulmonary artery dilatation, displacement due to lobar atelectasis.

Lungs

Overall and regional aeration, vascular dilatation, infiltrates, masses, cavities.

As you go scanning along, look especially for unusual sizes, contours and densities that cannot be explained sensibly on the basis of known anatomic considerations. After you have indulged your natural tendency to stare at the glaring abnormality on the film, move into an organized search pattern or check list.[6] If you skip that compulsive little technique and hop directly onto an obvious lung nodule, you may miss the subtle rib metastasis that completely alters the optimal management for your patient. As a double check before you stop searching, ask yourself, "Assuming a specific lesion, what additional findings should I seek that might be related to it?" For example, a peripheral pulmonary nodule (?cancer) should send you into a double check for hilar adenopathy, pleural effusion and bone destruction.

Describing and Communicating

A common frustration students often encounter is that they are perfectly able to see that something is abnormal on a film but have trouble describing and defining it. The "fruits and nuts" doctors employ terminology such as grapefruit-sized mass, apple-core colon carcinoma, sunburst bone lesion, boot-shaped heart and that infamous description of acute pulmonary edema, "a snowstorm in a birdcage." These terms may be quaint, comical or disgusting. Use them if you wish when they seem truly descriptive but realize that at times their imprecision may mislead you or distract you from thinking about the real pathology.

Here are some examples of "respectable" terms which may help you to describe what you see on abnormal chest films:

INFILTRATE

An abnormal pulmonary opacity with ill-defined margins. Its size, location and texture may permit some helpful conjecture regarding its nature.

EXAMPLE: "Localized patchy infiltrate, possibly excavated, posterior segment right upper lobe." That appearance would make you highly suspicious of active tuberculosis and alert you to isolate your patient while you try to isolate his organism.

NODULE OR MASS

Dense opacity which is rather sharply delineated from surrounding aerated lung. Tumors and granulomas are the commonest types.

LINEAR SCARRING

Dense, opaque linearities, often extending toward the pleura. These are left at the site of intense inflammation or ischemic necrosis. Coarse transverse lines at the lung bases may be scars or transitory foci of discoid or platelike atelectasis in a patient who is underventilating.

Mediastinum

Packed within the space bordered by lungs, sternum and spine are a large number of anatomically contiguous but functionally unrelated structures. The student who learned his anatomy in a "systems" orientation must now make an extra effort to integrate his knowledge. Mediastinal structures influence each other and are influenced as a group by pathologic processes. The effect of a large left atrium on the esophagus and left bronchus is one example. The manner in which esophageal carcinoma may erode into the trachea and also obstruct the superior vena cava is another.

Several factors assist us in evaluating the mediastinum. Its lateral borders are sharply seen at their interface with radiolucent lung, and the tracheal air column provides a lucent stripe of natural contrast down the center. If clinical circumstances or routine PA and lateral views raise suspicions, we can look at the mediastinum obliquely, fluoroscopically or tomographically. We have the technical capability to opacify all

Fig 2–2. – Mediastinal profiles in the midcoronal plane.

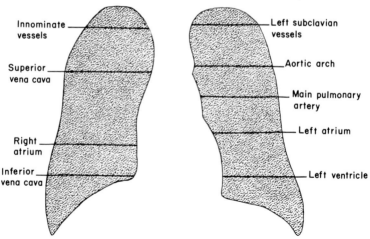

Innominate vessels

Superior vena cava

Right atrium

Inferior vena cava

Left subclavian vessels

Aortic arch

Main pulmonary artery

Left atrium

Left ventricle

of the mediastinum's hollow structures by means of angiography, bronchography and barium esophagography. Finally, we can infer things about radiologically invisible structures, as we do when we use diaphragmatic motion to assess the condition of the phrenic nerve.

Normal Radiographic Anatomy

Let us begin with the profiles readily appreciated in the coronal midplane.

Figure 2–2 is an accurate representation in an upright, vigorous 24-year-old medical student. His lusty 9-month-old son has an upper mediastinum filled with flabby, masslike thy-

Fig 2–3.—The mediastinum in depth. **A,** transverse section at T-4 level. **B,** transverse section at T-10. **C,** composite in frontal projection.

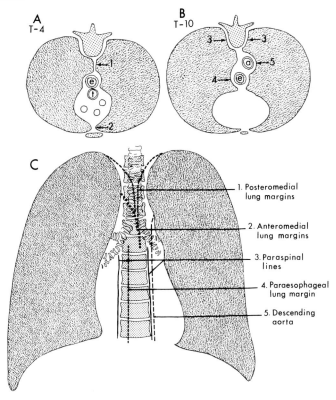

1. Posteromedial lung margins
2. Anteromedial lung margins
3. Paraspinal lines
4. Paraesophageal lung margin
5. Descending aorta

mus. His arteriosclerotic grandfather has calcification, elonga-
tion and tortuosity of the great vessels, bringing those structures into prominence as they bulge laterally out against aerated lung. Indeed, in some senescent chests this can lead to the
mistaken impression of right superior mediastinal mass. Finally, if the student is x-rayed while supine or in expiration, his
own mediastinum will be shortened and broadened into an
alarming appearance. Your developing baselines of normal
must take patient age and position into consideration.

Next let us probe the mediastinum a little more deeply, using a well-penetrated PA film[7] (Fig 2 – 3).

TRACHEAL AIR COLUMN

This column should be midline, except at the level of the
aortic arch, where it deviates slightly to the right.

MEDIAL LUNG MARGINS (Fig 2 – 3; profiles 1,2,4)

The medial edges of the lung are often visible through the
overlapping densities. Their normal location is assurance that
the mediastinum is not harboring a mass.

PARASPINAL LINES (Fig 2 – 3; profile 3)

These lines are the medial reflections of parietal pleura
along the spine. Vertebral tumor, hemorrhage and abscess can
cause these lines to bulge laterally.

DESCENDING AORTA (Fig 2 – 3; profile 5)

This is normally visible. Its configuration will vary with age,
showing a flat profile close to the spine in children and young
adults but later bowing laterally with senescent tortuosity. Its
margin will be obliterated by adjacent lower lobe or pleural
opacity.

Common Mediastinal Abnormalities

MEDIASTINAL EMPHYSEMA

In patients with obstructive pulmonary disease, air can rup-
ture from peripheral alveoli, track centrally within the lung

interstitium to the hilum and then enter the mediastinum. Chest trauma, endoscopy and violent vomiting are other potential causes of pneumomediastinum.

MEDIASTINAL MASSES

A wide variety of mass lesions can arise from the mediastinum. Etiologic categories include neoplastic, inflammatory, developmental, traumatic and degenerative. (That is not a bad way to organize thinking about pathology of any body region or system.) More helpful in contemplating the nature and significance of a given mass is to characterize its location (Fig 2–4). For embryologic reasons, certain lesions occur commonly in one locale and almost never in another area 5 cm away.

ANTERIOR. — Upper: thymoma, teratoma, thyroid mass, adenopathy, ascending aortic aneurysm. Lower: pericardial cyst, Morgagni hernia.

MIDDLE. — Aortic arch aneurysm, bronchogenic cyst, adenopathy, hiatus hernia, esophageal lesions.

POSTERIOR. — Neurogenic tumor, descending aortic aneurysm, adenopathy.

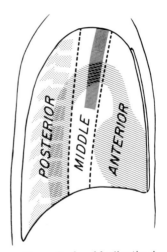

Fig   2–4. — Mediastinal compartments in lateral view.

The Cardiac Image

Chest films offer important information about cardiac structure and function to supplement your clinical and electrocardiographic data. Confident evaluation of the overall size and shape of the heart is certainly facilitated by the use of upright films, made in inspiration without significant rotation. As your experience and baselines broaden, however, portable films made in clinically distressed, technically compromised circumstances will also become comprehensible.

Cardiac Size

Most doctors "eyeball" the cardiac silhouette, judging its condition by reference to thousands of similar films that they have seen before. That is small comfort to a beginner. In the next refinement in quantitative efforts, the doctor jabs at the PA film with index and fifth fingers extended, using the interphalangeal distance as makeshift calipers. He is trying to

Fig 2–5. – Normal cardiac profiles. **A,** PA film. **B,** PA diagram. **C,** lateral film. **D,** lateral diagram.

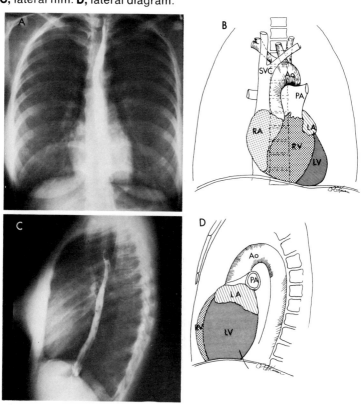

compare the transverse cardiac diameter to the width of the chest, knowing that in adults and older children the cardiac diameter is usually less than half the transverse thoracic diameter.

More precise measurements obviously exist, as do formulas and nomograms for relating calculated cardiac volume to body surface area. In selected instances these calculations can be very useful. More commonly you will find yourself having to compare current cardiac appearance with that recorded at a previous time. In addition to being sure that the geometric conditions of filming were comparable, you must be alert to the physiological variations in cardiac size and shape that oc-

Fig 2–6.—Normal cardiac profiles. **A,** right oblique film. **B,** right oblique diagram. **C,** left oblique film. **D,** left oblique diagram.

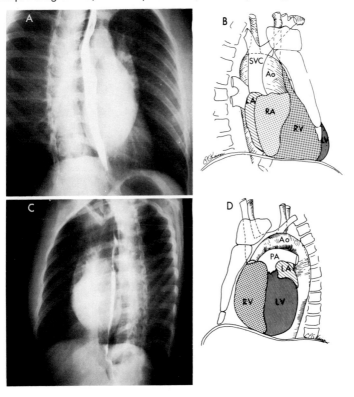

cur from moment to moment. Systole and diastole change the cardiac shape but affect the transverse cardiac diameter only slightly. Inadvertent respiratory maneuvers which vary intra-thoracic pressure and consequent venous return to the heart make measurable differences in cardiac diameter. Variations of 1 to 1.5 cm are not unusual. These transitory changes must be considered before an assumption is made concerning pathologic alteration in cardiac diameter since the previous examination.

The Cardiac Series

A sequence of diagnostic examinations of increasing complexity provide data of increasing specificity and accuracy. One step "up" from the standard chest films is the cardiac series, a four-view (PA, lateral, right and left obliques) examination made with barium in the esophagus. Again, normal relationships must be learned before pathologic variations can be perceived (Figs 2–5 and 2–6). Facts to be reviewed at this point include:

- the normal border-forming chambers on each view
- the expected location of mitral and aortic valves, to facilitate later searches for calcification
- the relationship of each chamber to other mediastinal structures

Students are often uneasy with spatial orientation on oblique films. A rapid cure is to watch several chest fluoroscopies and spend a few minutes rotating an anatomic heart model. It then becomes evident that the cardiac shape is very different on the two obliques: elongated in the right oblique and foreshortened or "apex-on" in the left oblique. For rapid orientation, if you are fumbling the films onto viewboxes during Grand Rounds, keep the gastric bubble on the patient's left.

The oblique projections occasionally provide unique information concerning some aspect of the cardiac contour but more often simply confirm impressions extracted from the PA and lateral views.

Chamber Analysis

In congestive heart failure and the cardiomyopathies, diffuse multichamber enlargement is generally present. Rheumatic valvular disease and congenital heart lesions, however, usually do show specific chamber predominance. Although it must be reluctantly acknowledged that one *grossly* enlarged chamber can displace normal chambers into misleading profiles, there are predictable contours of selective chamber enlargement which can be relied upon and should be learned (Fig 2–7 and 2–8).

Pericardial Effusion

Any time you are confronted by a large cardiac silhouette, consider the possibility that pericardial effusion rather than actual cardiomegaly might be responsible. This is particularly appropriate if the pulmonary vasculature appears too normal or if the "heart" has enlarged quickly. Although texts describe a characteristic "water bottle" shape in PA view, a dilated, failing heart can achieve that same distinction. In lateral projection it is sometimes possible to identify the thin lucent stripe of fat on the epicardial surface. If this is displaced from the substernal fat, pericardial fluid is interposed.

Chest fluoroscopy will show "dampened" pulsations, because the radiologist is watching the fluid-filled pericardium and not the myocardium. The epicardial fat lucency is more often detectable fluoroscopically. If it is displaced from the external silhouette, differentiation of effusion from poorly contractile myocardium can be made.

A few years ago angiocardiography would have been the next procedure "up" if chest films and fluoroscopy failed to provide definitive diagnosis. Subsequently, a radionuclide technique emerged providing imaging of the blood pool within the chambers which could then be compared to the external radiographic image. A substantial discrepancy indicated pericardial effusion or enormously hypertrophied myocardium.

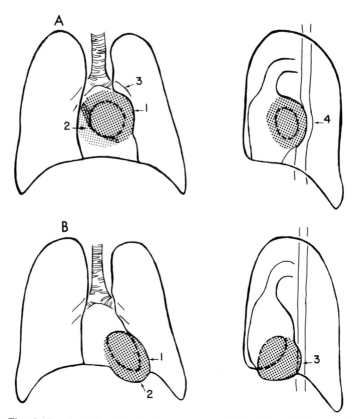

Fig 2–7.—A, left atrial enlargement: (1) bulging left auricular appendage, (2) double density seen through right atrium, (3) elevated left main bronchus, (4) posterior esophageal displacement. **B,** left ventricular enlargement: (1) enlarges to left, (2) downward, (3) posteriorly.

Currently, however, echocardiography is the procedure of choice. In a simple, innocuous, relatively inexpensive procedure, ultrasound waves can be deflected from posterior myocardial and pericardial surfaces and an abnormal intervening distance can be accurately perceived. Figure 2–9 shows a patient with a pericardial effusion before and after pericardiocentesis. At the time of the tap, air was introduced so that the pericardium could be examined for tumor nodules.

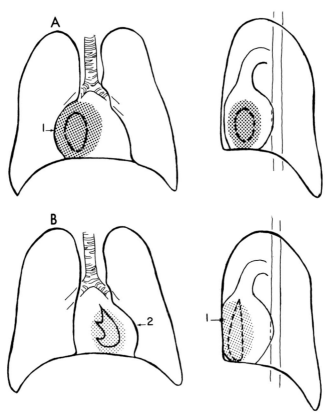

Fig 2–8.–**A,** right atrial enlargement: (1) bulging right heart border, a difficult "call." **B,** right ventricular enlargement: (1) full retrosternal space on lateral projection, (2) RV enlargement, if great enough, elevates apex of left ventricle.

The Pulmonary Vasculature

Study of the pulmonary vessels will provide you with a very meaningful gauge of your patient's hemodynamic status. There are well-established[8] patterns of vascular dilatation, constriction and distribution that inform you of existing flows and pressures. This information helps you sort out congenital and acquired heart disease and warns you of impending heart failure before other signs are clear-cut. Again, a very sound

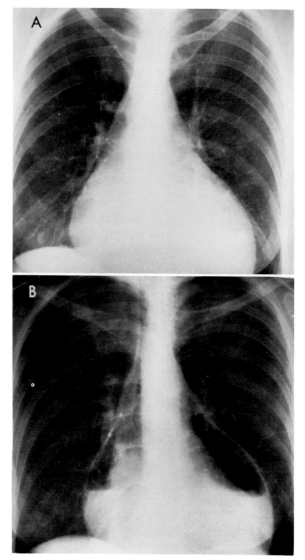

Fig 2–9.—A, large pericardial effusion; **B,** fluid partially removed; air injected. Note huge cardiac silhouette with normal pulmonary vasculature.

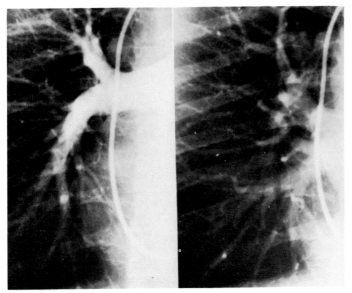

Fig 2–10.—Pulmonary arteriogram showing arterial and venous phases. Note differences in location and direction of lower lobe vessels, gradual tapering from central to peripheral vessels.

grip on normal appearances is vital. You need to take every opportunity to view large numbers of chest films in patients without cardiovascular disease. The vessels *are* readily visible now that you are paying attention to them. You need to be aware of a normal baseline, or all vasculature will look "prominent" to you. For emphasis and anatomic review, refer to Figure 2–10, which shows the arterial and venous phases of a pulmonary arteriogram. Note the branching patterns, the vessel size centrally and peripherally, the caliber of upper and lower lobe vessels and the difference in slope of the lower lobe arteries and veins. Figures 2–11 and 2–12 present, in a deliberately exaggerated form, the basic patterns of altered hemodynamics.

A. Normal

In the upright position the upper lobe vessels are distinctly smaller in caliber than those at the bases. In addition, the central vessels taper gradually as they branch to the periphery.

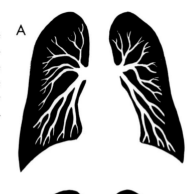

B. Increased Flow

All of the vessels — central and peripheral, upper and lower — are proportionally dilated.

CAUSES

- left to right shunt — septal defect, patent ductus
- high output states — severe anemia, thyrotoxicosis

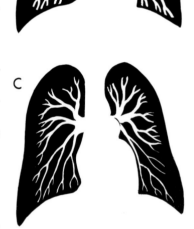

C. Pulmonary Venous Congestion

(pulmonary venous hypertension)

The upper lobe vessels are selectively dilated.

CAUSES

- mitral stenosis
- failing left ventricle
- atrial myxoma

Note: This is the first step in the congestive failure pattern to be described later.

Fig 2–11. — Pulmonary vasculature. **A,** normal. **B,** increased flow. **C,** pulmonary venous congestion.

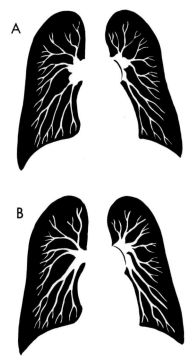

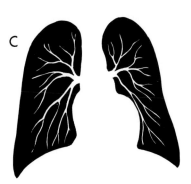

A. Pulmonary Arterial Hypertension

The central arteries bulge and then abruptly narrow to small peripheral branches.

CAUSES
- chronic pulmonary disease
- recurrent pulmonary emboli
- long-standing flow or pressure increase

B. Poststenotic Dilatation

Turbulent flow distal to pulmonic valvular stenosis weakens and dilates the main and left pulmonary arteries. The right pulmonary artery often remains of normal size.

C. Diminished Flow

Lung vessels—central and peripheral, upper and lower—are of diminished caliber.

CAUSES
- some forms of cyanotic congenital heart disease, including tetralogy of Fallot and tricuspid atresia.

Fig 2–12.—Pulmonary vasculature *(cont.)* **A,** pulmonary arterial hypertension. **B,** poststenotic dilatation. **C,** diminished flow.

Left Heart Failure

The chest findings in heart failure are best understood as a sequence of pathophysiologic events. If failure occurs slowly, each step may be visible; if precipitously, then the phases may telescope and overlap.

DILATATION OF UPPER LOBE VESSELS

In the upright normal patient, upper lobe vessels are visibly *smaller* than those in the lower lobes. However, when left atrial pressure reaches about 25 mm of mercury, lower lobe vessels constrict, more right ventricular output is diverted to the upper lobes, and the vessel caliber there increases. The veins are more visibly affected than are the arteries.

INTERSTITIAL EDEMA

As left atrial pressures continue to rise, transudation of fluid occurs into the lung interstitium, thickening the alveolar walls and interlobular connective tissues. This results in multiple *linear* densities first described by Kerley and designated alphabetically.

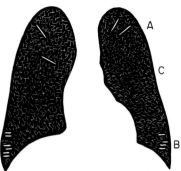

A lines are long, nonbranching linear densities, obliquely directed to the hilum.

B lines are short, thin transverse lines best seen laterally near the costophrenic angles.

C lines are fine reticular meshwork, the result of multiple overlapping lines.

Note: The "B" lines have achieved the most popularity. They all have the same significance.

Fig 2–13. — Interstitial pulmonary edema.

In patients with chronic or recurrent failure, the interstitial connective tissue thickens and becomes capable of trapping more fluid than is the case with normal lungs. Well-developed

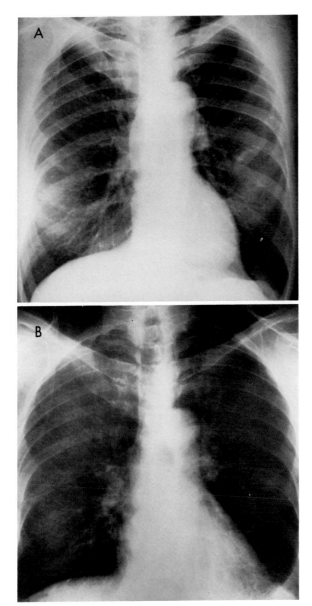

Fig 2–14.—Aortic valvular disease. **A,** compensated. **B,** in failure. Note cardiac enlargement, vascular engorgement and pleural effusion.

Kerley lines are therefore more likely to be encountered in a patient with long-standing mitral stenosis than in someone whose first episode of failure has just been precipitated by an acute myocardial infarction.[9]

INTRA-ALVEOLAR EDEMA

Continued transudation progresses to actual outpouring of fluid into alveolar spaces. Ill-defined, coalescent opacities spread outwards, usually symmetrically. With replacement of air by fluid, the images of distended vessels and edematous interstitium are lost. This is the stage at which abnormal physical findings may first become apparent. Keep in mind that the "classic" appearance of cardiogenic pulmonary edema:

- may be asymmetric if patient was lying on one side before filming or has patchy emphysema
- may be edema of another etiology (renal failure, smoke inhalation, acute heroin intoxication)
- may not be edema fluid at all (but may be pneumonia or hemorrhage)

Figure 2–14 shows a patient with aortic valvular disease when well-compensated and later in heart failure. Note development of parenchymal opacities, vascular engorgement, pleural effusions and increased cardiomegaly.

Right Heart Failure

When right atrial pressures increase, the effects of systemic venous hypertension may be evident radiologically:

1. Dilated azygos vein. This should not be much bigger than 7 mm in upright non-pregnant adult.
2. Convex, bulging inferior vena cava profile. Normally this should be straight or concave.
3. Pleural fluid.
4. High diaphragm, due to large liver, ascites.

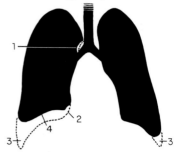

Fig 2–15. — Right heart failure.

It is obviously beyond the scope of this manual to progress much further into cardiac radiology. Simple filming techniques and analyses fall into the category of preliminary assessment which supplements clinical and basic laboratory data. When these point to the probability of correctable disease such as malformations, valvular scarring or coronary artery disease, more definitive information is required. Cardiac catheterization, angiocardiography and echocardiography, for precise physiologic and morphologic detail, then provide the cardiologist and cardiac surgeon with the completed evaluation.

Abnormalities of the Pleura

Pneumothorax

This is a condition you must learn to recognize. You will see it following spontaneous blowout of a bleb, major chest trauma with lung laceration, lung puncture and leak incurred during thoracentesis or lung biopsy. If the pneumothorax is small, there may be no physical signs, and you will have to rely entirely upon the chest film.

A small pneumothorax will appear as a strip of radiolucency, external to the visceral pleural surface and devoid of vascular markings (Fig 2–16, A). Upright filming is ideal. You would look for air over the apex and along the lateral portion of the upper lobe. An expiratory phase film will sometimes show it when inspiratory filming is equivocal.

Supine filming is likely to miss all but the very large pneumothoraces. Air is layered under the anterior chest wall and may not cast a visible image. Any suggestions for the patient who cannot assume the upright position?*

A variation on this problem is the "pseudopneumothorax" caused by a skin wrinkle superimposed on the chest, simulating the visceral pleural line. Detection of lung markings lateral to the line solves that problem.

---

*Lateral decubitus—patient rolled onto his unaffected side; film taken with horizontal beam to show air between visceral and parietal pleura on the "up" side.

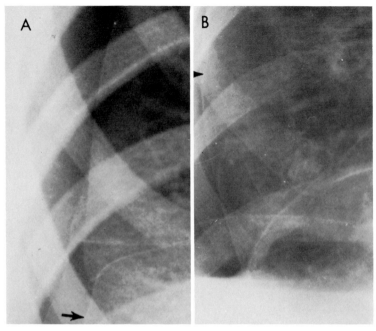

Fig 2–16.—Air in pleural space. **A,** pneumothorax. **B,** hydropneumothorax. Arrows show visceral pleural surface.

Tension Pneumothorax

If there is a "flutter valve" effect and the intrapleural pressure increases, the mediastinum will begin to shift. Vascular and ventilatory compromise may occur quickly and require emergency decompression.

Pleural Effusion

When you are searching for pleural fluid, several facts concerning its distribution often prove useful.

The posterior costophrenic recess is deeper than the lateral

SMALL PLEURAL EFFUSION

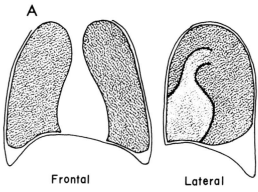

A

Frontal   Lateral

VERY SMALL PLEURAL EFFUSION

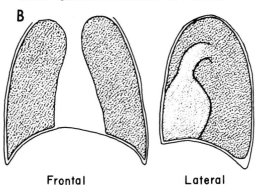

B

Frontal   Lateral

Fig 2–17.—Detection of **A,** small and **B,** very small pleural effusions.

Fig 2–18.—Subpulmonic pleural effusions.

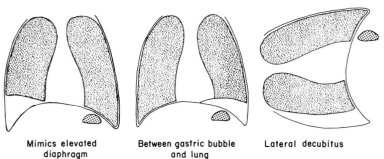

Mimics elevated diaphragm

Between gastric bubble and lung

Lateral decubitus

INTERLOBAR EFFUSION

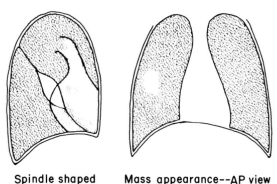

Spindle shaped   Mass appearance--AP view
Fig 2–19. – Interlobar effusion.

one; therefore in the upright position a very small effusion is best seen in lateral projection (Fig 2 – 17).

Subpulmonic pleural effusion may accumulate between the diaphragm and the undersurface of the lung in the upright position (Fig 2 – 18). On the left side, this will show as a soft tissue space between aerated lung and gastric air bubble. On the right, it can mimic an elevated diaphragm. In either case, a lateral decubitus film with the affected side *down* will clarify the diagnosis as the fluid rolls out into a visible position along the lateral chest wall.

Interlobar effusion. Fluid lurking in a fissure can be mistaken for a lung mass on AP projection. A lateral view, however, shows the characteristic location and biconvex configuration (Fig 2 – 19). There are usually, but not always, other evidences of pleural abnormality.

Hydropneumothorax. When a pleural effusion has a perfectly flat rather than a laterally upcurved surface, suspect coexistent pleural air (Fig 2 – 16, B).

The Pulmonary Hila

Normally the "hilar shadows" on chest x-rays are formed almost entirely by the pulmonary vessels. The bronchi are air-

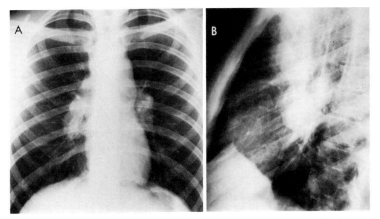

Fig 2–20.—Hilar and mediastinal adenopathy. **A,** PA. **B,** lateral projections.

filled and thin walled and cause little opacity. The lymph nodes are small and flat, presenting negligible profiles.

One of the causes of hilar enlargement is dilatation of the pulmonary arteries because of increased arterial pressure.

Unilateral hilar mass is a common presentation for bronchogenic carcinoma. That finding should incite prompt, aggressive workup, beginning with sputum cytologies and including bronchoscopy.

Bilateral hilar masses are usually due to adenopathy and may be accompanied by adenopathy in the mediastinum. The leading differential considerations here are lymphoma, sarcoidosis and tuberculosis (Fig. 2–20).

The Lung Parenchyma

Infiltrates — Predominantly Alveolar

DEFINITION

Processes which flood the alveolar air spaces with fluid or cells produce "soft," patchy, confluent, ill-defined lung densities. Pneumonia, edema, hemorrhage and some forms of tumor are examples.

Recognition

Some pulmonary infiltrates are dense, large and conveniently placed in areas where not even the patient can fail to see them when you point them out. Others cause more subtle images but are no less important to detect.

Location may be the problem, as in a posteromedial lower lobe opacity, hiding behind the heart on PA view and over the spine on lateral. Lesions in the apices may be sheltered by ribs and clavicles, while central lesions may be lost in the confusion of vascular shadows. Other abnormalities are of only modest density or have wispy edges without eye-catching demarcations. Some of these abnormalities are more obvious when viewed from a few feet away or with the use of a minifying lens.

Certain useful signs have emerged to aid in the detection of more ambiguous infiltrates. Air-filled bronchi become visible when they are surrounded by infiltrated, consolidated tissue. This has been called the *air bronchogram* sign by Felson.[27] It may help you to spot a subtle infiltrate hidden behind the heart, for instance. An infiltrate is not very photogenic in that location; Figure 2–21 shows one in a more accessible place.

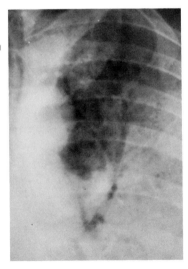

Fig 2–21.—Air bronchogram in pulmonary consolidation.

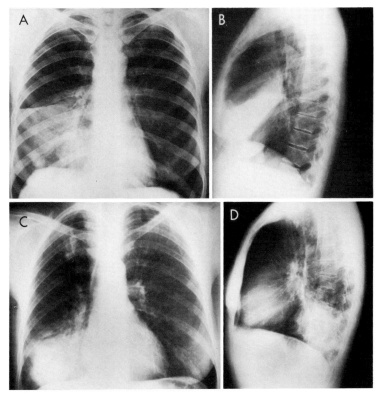

Fig 2–22.—Lobar pneumonia patients. Patient #1, **A** and **B.** Patient #2, **C** and **D.**

Another helper in recognizing small infiltrates has been dubbed the *silhouette sign*. Normally the profiles of the heart, the mediastinum and the diaphragm are visible because a tissue of different density, i.e., aerated lung, is up against them. If that bit of lung becomes infiltrated with water-density pus or blood, the silhouette or visible edge is lost. Figure 2–22 shows two patients, both with lobar consolidation. Can you differentiate middle from lower lobe involvement on the PA film? Was your detection of the additional *upper* lobe infiltrate in the lower lobe pneumonia patient delayed by your preoccupation with the right heart border?

Interpretation

We can offer fairly sensible suggestions regarding the nature of an alveolar infiltrate by considering its distribution, evolution, associated radiologic features and clinical setting.[28] Guesses regarding the specific agent responsible for a pneumonia become more tenuous and simply play with statistical probabilities. Tuberculosis has a greater tendency to excavate than certain other diseases, viral pneumonias are less likely to be lobar. These speculations are always interesting, but obviously definitive laboratory confirmation is needed.

Infiltrates — Predominantly Interstitial

Certain pathologic processes which predominantly involve the interstitial pulmonary tissues and tend to spare the alveoli produce a nonconfluent linear or very finely granular pattern. The lines may be arranged transversely, or they may interdigitate to produce a "honeycombed" appearance. The infiltrating material may be fibrous (pneumoconiosis or collagen disease), edematous (the pre-alveolar phase of heart failure), neoplastic (permeation by metastatic neoplasm) or inflammatory.

The pattern itself is nonspecific, and problem solving re-

Fig 2–23.—Fibrosis and pulmonary arterial hypertension due to eosinophilic granuloma.

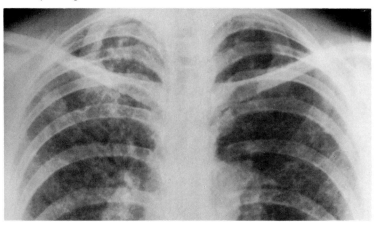

quires close correlation of clinical and radiologic features. Associated radiologic findings such as hilar adenopathy, cardiomegaly or pleural abnormality could give clues to the basis for the interstitial process. For example, a rare disease, eosinophilic granuloma of lung (a reticuloendotheliosis), evolves into a honeycombed pattern of scarring and blebs (Fig. 2–23), may go on to pulmonary hypertension and can cause pneumothorax. Similarly a history of occupational exposure, multisystem disease or antecedent tumor would have obvious implications. Lung biopsy is sometimes required and usually, but not always, is definitive.[29]

Atelectasis

SUBSEGMENTAL, DISCOID OR PLATE-LIKE ATELECTASIS

Coarse transverse linear densities at the lung bases are frequently seen in patients who are breathing shallowly. These are often the *result* of severe chest or abdominal pain and should not be misinterpreted as the cause.

LOBAR ATELECTASIS

Collapse will predictably occur following occlusion of a lobar bronchus. You can also predict that if it is not recognized and corrected, infection, fibrosis and permanent lobar damage may ensue.

Direct signs include displaced fissures, crowded vessels, crowded air-bronchograms and increased lobar density. Subtle changes in lobar density are best detected by a careful comparison with the opposite side. In some instances the density difference may be enhanced if you deliberately blur your vision to minimize distracting details of ribs and vessels. "Blurrograms" may be created by ptosis of glasses or eyelids.

Indirect signs may be more obvious. Look for compensatory mediastinal shift, diaphragmatic elevation, crowded ribs and overexpansion of other lobes (Fig. 2–24).

Etiologies include endobronchial obstruction by tumor, mucus plugs or aspirated foreign material. Another possible

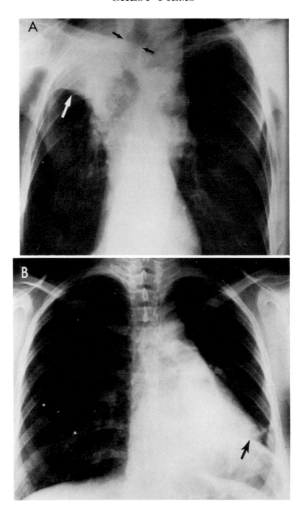

Fig 2–24.–Lobar atelectasis with compensatory shifts. **A,** right upper lobe. **B,** left lower lobe.

cause is extrinsic bronchial compression; adenopathy can affect the right middle lobe and gross left atrial enlargement can affect the left lower lobe.

CHECK-VALVE OBSTRUCTIONS

Aspirated foreign bodies may permit air to enter a lobe but cause obstruction during expiration when bronchial caliber is less. The result is air-trapping, best seen by a comparison of expiratory and inspiratory films. Figure 2–25 is an x-ray film of a toddler who prowled the rug after a cocktail party. Note the mediastinal shift.

Emphysema

It is essential to appreciate both the limitations and the specific usefulness of chest x-rays in the diagnosis of obstructive pulmonary disease.[10] There is a group of patients with severe obstruction and only modest overexpansion whose chest films look quite innocuous despite profound physiological impairment.

The radiologic signs of large lung volumes—increased AP chest diameter, low diaphragms and very radiolucent lungs—simply duplicate your findings on physical examination. You can better use the chest film to seek localized bullae, peribronchial infiltrates and abnormal air collections in the pleural space or mediastinum.

The pulmonary vasculature in emphysema merits additional attention. As mentioned previously, radiographic evidence of pulmonary arterial hypertension (i.e., bulging central hilar arteries) may be present. In addition, in areas where overinflation and destruction of parenchyma are prominent, the vessels are displaced and attenuated. Most of the pulmonary circulation is diverted to more normal areas, making those areas *appear* hypervascular and dense. For instance, if bullous changes predominate in the lung bases, flow is diverted to the upper zones, simulating the pattern of pulmonary venous congestion (hypertension). If a patient with irregularly distributed patches of emphysema goes into left heart failure and

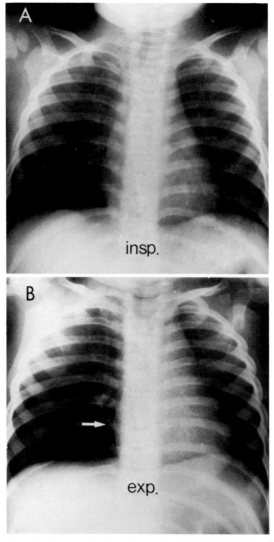

Fig 2–25.—Aspirated foreign body in right bronchus. **A,** inspiratory film. **B,** expiratory film showing marked hyperaeration on right with mediastinal shift.

pulmonary edema, the normally vascularized lung becomes edematous and the bullous areas are spared. The patchiness of the edema could be misleading.

Pulmonary Embolus

Pathologists tell us that an astoundingly high incidence of pulmonary arterial thrombi is found on autopsies of hospitalized patients. The clinician and radiologist must have a very high index of suspicion and an awareness that the much advertised presentation of chest pain, hemoptysis and triangular pulmonary density is, in fact, unusual.

Several radiologic features *may* be present singly or in combination. These include pleural fluid, parenchymal densities, slight diaphragmatic elevation, distended hilar vessels and hypovascular peripheral lung segments. None of these need to be present, however, and sometimes the chest film is absolutely *negative.*

If you are suspicious of an embolus, do not let a negative chest x-ray dissuade you from requesting a more definitive examination. The *radionuclide perfusion lung scan* is a reasonably accurate indicator of lung perfusion and will often furnish the definitive answer.

You should be aware of some basic limitations to the accuracy of this type of scan. Remember that patients with areas of obstructive emphysema have diminished perfusion in those areas, which appear as "cold" areas, simulating pulmonary emboli. By comparing radioactive gas ventilation scans with the perfusion scan pattern, you can avoid that mistake. The second common problem is the scan which is positive in an area that is abnormally dense on x-ray. Pneumonia can cause that finding just as readily as infarction. However, additional perfusion scan defects in areas where the x-ray is negative provide good evidence for emboli.

If the scans are equivocal and major management decisions (anticoagulation, vena caval plication, etc.) require a definitive answer, pulmonary arteriography is indicated.

Figure 2–26 shows a patient with abnormality at the left base on chest x-ray; the arteriogram and scan show gross oc-

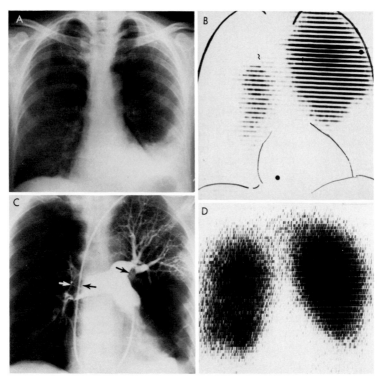

Fig 2–26. – Massive pulmonary emboli. **A,** PA chest showing left basilar opacity. **B,** perfusion scan showing huge defect on right as well as at left base. **C,** pulmonary arteriogram showing large filling defects *(arrows).* **D,** perfusion scan immediately following embolectomies.

clusion and nonperfusion on the *right* as well as the expected abnormality in the left lower lobe. Embolectomy was performed.

Tuberculosis

This is a bad disease for the patient but a good one for use in reviewing a wide gamut of chest x-ray appearances. Depending upon the stage of disease and the response of the patient, intrathoracic tuberculosis can show:

● Apical infiltration. The caseating excavating stage is frequently seen in the apices, partially obscured by overlapping ribs and clavicles. Apical lordotic views angulate upward to achieve a "bone free" look at the apex. If that is unsuccessful, body section tomography can blur out overlying planes and "focus" on the lesion.

- Pleural effusion. This occasionally is massive, especially in primary infection.
- Hilar adenopathy. This often is striking, even without visible parenchymal disease.
- Calcified primary complex. There is a calcified focus in the lung and in the draining hilar node.
- Miliary dissemination. Film shows innumerable tiny nodules. If the patient survives, these granulomas become fibrotic and may calcify.
- Endobronchial stenosis and atelectasis. Bronchography is occasionally required to delineate the site of obstruction.

Supplementary Procedures in Chest Radiology

Several supplementary procedures in chest radiology that apply to specific disease processes and their diagnosis have already been mentioned:

radionuclide lung scans
pulmonary arteriogram
lateral decubitus filming
expiratory filming
tomography
apical lordotic projection
bronchography

To illustrate the role of others let us consider another frequent clinical problem, the solitary pulmonary nodule (alias "coin lesion").

Case Report

At your office one morning you see Mr. Johansen, a 60-year-old truck driver who has had a postnasal drip and smoker's "hack" for years. He feels well and has not seen a doctor in three years but comes in now, at his wife's urging, for a check-up. Physical examination is normal, but you conclude your data collection by sending him to have a chest x-ray. The radiologist calls you back immediately to report a "1.5 cm nodule in the posterior segment of the right upper lobe, 4 cm away from the hilum. There is no visible adenopathy, pleural effusion or bone metastasis." What do you do next?

One approach would be immediate thoracotomy. A frozen section in the operating room would determine whether wedge resection of the nodule or major lobectomy should be performed. If he has a carcinoma, your patient has been given every possible chance for survival. If the nodule is only a healed granuloma, the mortality and morbidity risks of thoracotomy are probably inappropriate.

Another approach would be to tell your patient, "You have a spot on your lung. It is really quite small, and you have probably had it for years. We'll take another x-ray in three months, and if the spot is changing, we'll look into it." If three months later the nodule *has* grown, that delay may have cost the patient his chance for resection before lymphatic spread.

I hope you are persuaded that your decision should be immediate investigation of the nodule. Although it is likely that the nodule is either a primary carcinoma or an old granuloma, other possibilities include arteriovenous malformation, hamartoma, metastatic carcinoma or an old scar from an infarct or hematoma. Where do you begin a workup and how far do you go?

The single most important thing that you can do to begin sorting out these possibilities is to *locate a previous chest film.* It is possible but unlikely that the patient has never been filmed before. He may have been x-rayed in another city or in conjunction with something nonmemorable like an insurance or employment physical or a health department mobile x-ray survey. If you can examine a previous film you can find out how long the patient has had the lesion. This may settle the problem; i.e., a long-term, absolutely stable nodule is a scar of some kind, and nothing need be done about it. If that is the case, be thorough in your explanation and reassurances and do not leave the patient with lingering anxiety.

If a film made a few years ago did not show the nodule, then investigation should be continued. Your clinical evaluation should, of course, be meticulous. Findings such as peripheral adenopathy, an abdominal mass, hepatomegaly or blood in the urine sediment or stool may be related to the x-ray abnormality and should be investigated by clinical and radiologic means.

If these findings are absent, attention can be centered on the chest. Many clinicans would perform tuberculin and fungus *skin tests*. But in this particular case, little may be gained. A negative result would maintain and intensify your concern, but you are already pretty worried. A positive skin test should *not* reassure you. It may be totally unrelated to the suspicious lesion. It is reasonable to examine the patient's sputum for malignant cells, but the percentage positive yield on sputum cytology from relatively peripheral malignant nodules is disappointing.

The radiologic examinations potentially pertinent to your workup should be considered in two categories.

ASSESSING THE NATURE OF THE LESION

This group of examinations is aimed at determining the etiology of the lesion. This began with the original description of it and included comparison with older films. It could involve fluoroscopic assessment for pulsation and tomographic scrutiny for calcification. In this regard you should realize that only well-formed, concentric calcification can be assumed to be granulomatous. A small fleck is nonspecific. Most significantly, however, in this first group of studies the radiologist can often obtain a small but diagnostic tissue specimen.

Percutaneous Lung Biopsy. — Under fluoroscopic control the lesion is localized, a long thin needle is inserted, and a core or aspirate of material is obtained for histologic and bacteriologic study. One third of patients develop a small pneumothorax, but these seldom require pleural aspiration or catheter. A theoretical risk of "seeding" malignant cells along the needle tract does exist. However, in several very large series, this did not, in fact, occur.[6]

Transbronchial Brushing. — During fluoroscopic monitoring a thin, opaque, controllable catheter is inserted transbronchially and manipulated through the bronchial tree into close proximity to the lesion. Gentle motion of a fine wire brush is then used to dislodge cells for cytologic evaluation.

ASSESSING RESECTABILITY

The second group of radiologic evaluations attempts to assess the potential resectability of a lesion already proved to be malignant. Metastatic nodes in the mediastinum predict a grim prognosis.

Chest Fluoroscopy. — Phrenic nerve invasion visibly impairs diaphragmatic motion. Deviation of the barium-filled esophagus occurs in the presence of subcarinal adenopathy.

Angiography. — Pulmonary arteriography may show compression or even obstruction of a pulmonary artery by adjacent or invasive tumor. This generally implies that the lesion is not resectable.

Computed tomography of the mediastinum has become increasingly accurate, and it complements mediastinoscopy in assessing regional spread of tumor.

Preoperative assessment would include a search for distant metastases, in view of the aggressiveness of many pulmonary neoplasms. It would probably include radionuclide scans of liver and bone and possibly brain.

CASE REPORT — FOLLOW-UP

Mr. Johansen had had a negative chest x-ray four years ago. His current workup included negative sputum cytologies and a positive second strength tuberculin test. Percutaneous lung biopsy was performed and yielded adenocarcinoma cells. Fluoroscopy, bronchoscopy and mediastinoscopy were negative. Tomography, angiography and bronchography were considered and discarded as unlikely to provide decision-altering information in this particular case. Mr. Johansen underwent right upper lobectomy, and at the time of surgery no adenopathy or pleural involvement was detected. The tumor was a moderately well-differentiated adenocarcinoma. This was three years ago; he is currently well, and there is reason for cautious optimism.

3

SKELETAL RADIOLOGY

X-RAY EXAMINATIONS often constitute a critically important part of your overall evaluation of patients with disease or injury of the skeletal system. Radiographic features that can lead to prompt diagnosis and appropriate treatment are present in a wide variety of traumatic, inflammatory, neoplastic and metabolic diseases.[31]. At times these findings simply support a moderately firm clinical diagnosis; in other cases, however, the films may provide the only clues to a clinically obscure situation. The diligence and skill of the observer determine whether these clues are perceived or disregarded.

An organized system of film analysis is as important here as it is for the chest film.

Study Method

Preliminary Overview

Get oriented; do not plunge into detail yet. Be sure you are certain of the body part and of the view from which you are seeing it. Filming of living patients occasionally results in views and images that are not immediately familiar. Careful attempts to portray extremities in traditional views may be thwarted by clinical circumstances of pain, limitation of motion, bulky dressings or altered states of consciousness.

Assess the adequacy of radiographic techniques. Dark, overexposed films penetrate dense structures well but "burn out" the soft tissues. Some information is retrievable with very bright illuminators (film melters). An underexposed or light film shows the soft tissues very well but may fail to provide

53

good bone images. We have no tricks to compensate for that problem. Finally, note whether the image is sharp or whether it is blurred by motion.

Soft Tissues

Study these areas carefully, seeking specific abnormalities.

FINDINGS	SIGNIFICANCE
Muscle wasting	Disuse paralysis, primary muscle disease
Soft tissue swelling	Hemorrhage, traumatic edema, inflammation, venous or lymphatic stasis
Calcifications	Old trauma, chronic venous stasis, metabolic, parasitic or connective tissue disorders
Opaque foreign bodies	Precise spatial localization required for removal
Gas in tissue planes	Penetrating trauma, infection by gas-forming bacteria
Adjacent surprises	Unsuspected renal calculi on spine films of a patient with back pain

Bone Shape and Size

Analysis of the configuration of the bone and its relationship to other bones is needed at this point. This is the step in which you will detect or exclude fractures, dislocations, congenital anomalies and acquired deformities.

Bone Surfaces

As you study the sharp interface between cortical bone and the adjacent soft tissues, look specifically for the following:

Periosteal New Bone Formation. — This is visible as a linear *density* closely paralleling the cortex. It may be a localized response to trauma, tumor or infection, as the periosteum lays down bone in response to its dissection by blood, malignant cells, pus or edema. In a more generalized form this is termed "hypertrophic pulmonary osteoarthropathy." It can accompany nail-bed "clubbing" and is a clue to intrathoracic neoplasm or suppuration. The pathogenesis of this phenomenon is obscure, but the end result is subperiosteal edema and consequent bone formation. Healing scurvy, hypervitaminosis A and D and infantile cortical hyperostosis (Caffey's disease) are possibilities if the patient is a child.

Juxta-articular Erosions. — These are focal, marginated cortical defects seen in arthritis.

Diffuse Cortical Resorption. — In hyperparathyroidism, bone resorption results in a smudgy, irregular loss of cortical integrity along the diaphysis of the phalanges.

Internal Structure

The search at this stage is for generalized alteration in mineralization, an abnormally altered texture, or foci of localized destruction.

Now that your overall analysis is completed, return to the specific clinical question and recheck that point. A localized physical finding or subjective complaint warrants a directed, intensified scrutiny.

Skeletal Trauma

In caring for patients with injured extremities, and before tackling the mechanical problems of fracture reduction, pause a moment to consider the potential likelihood of significant soft tissue injury. You need to think about the possibility of neurovascular damage, capsular and ligamentous tears, hemarthroses and invisible cartilage injury. Your clinical evaluation of these possibilities may, in selected instances, be helped by:

- stress views to test ligamentous stability
- contralateral views to compare epiphyseal appearance
- arteriography where major arterial injury is a serious consideration

Initial X-ray Evaluation of the Fracture

General Considerations

Several factors will significantly influence the prognosis for healing and your choice of management. Before assessing the geometric relationships at a fracture site, ask yourself:

- Does the fracture enter a joint? Is the growth plate damaged? Is the local vascularity in jeopardy?
- Is there complete disruption or just greenstick buckling? Is the fracture impacted and stable? Did it occur through previously pathologic bone?

Geometric Arrangements at a Fracture Site

The kinds of relationships illustrated in Figure 3–1 are readily perceived when frontal and lateral views of a fracture are viewed. *Rotation* of the distal fragment along its longitudinal axis can be subtler. Radiologic assessment requires seeing the full length of the bone and ascertaining that its proximal and distal anatomic landmarks "line up."

Ten commonly encountered fractures are shown in Figures 3–2 and 3–3. Describe them and contemplate their mechanisms and implications before checking your answers (on p. 155).

Fig 3–1.—Arrangements at a fracture site. **A,** greenstick. **B,** displaced. **C,** angulated. **D,** overriding. **E,** distracted. **F,** comminuted.

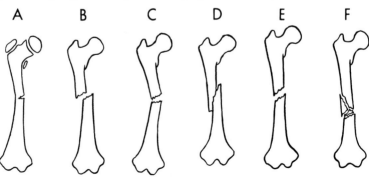

A   B   C   D   E   F

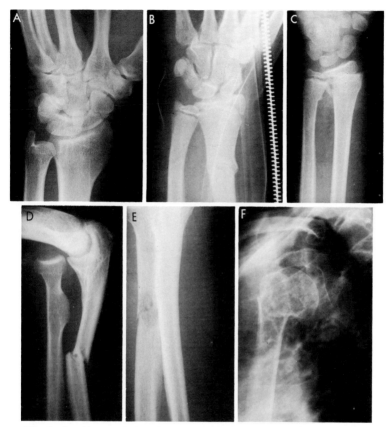

Fig 3–2.—Upper extremity fractures **A–F**. (Answer key on page 155.)

Role of X-ray Studies in Management and Followup

POSTREDUCTION FILMS

After external manipulation or operative reduction of the fracture, films are taken to check the alteration. Clinical factors in a given case determine whether the goal is anatomic perfection or early mobility. The "adequacy" of reduction can be judged only in this light. In some instances aggressive reduction and prolonged immobilization can lead to pericapsular

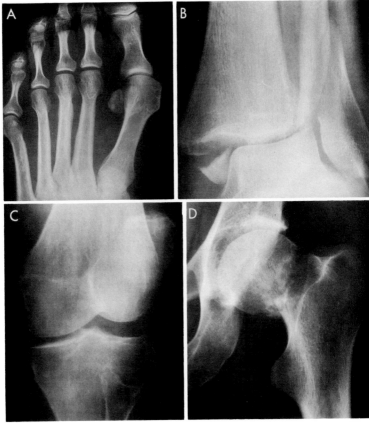

Fig 3–3. — Lower extremity fractures **A–D**. (Answer key on page 155.)

soft tissue scarring and serious functional impairment. Beautiful x-rays would be little consolation to patients in those cases.

FOLLOWUP FILMS IN PLASTER

As you would anticipate, knowing that a plaster cast is made of $CaSO_4$, image quality on followup films is poor; both fracture and early callus are frequently obscured. The purpose of the films, however, is primarily to check maintenance of alignment, and this is generally possible. It should be emphasized that, as you view a sequence of followup films, relatively minor variations in positioning will alter apparent relationships at a fracture site. Slight obliquity, for instance, will change the image substantially if there is displacement or angulation. You will not be misled into thinking that you have "lost" the good reduction, however, if you recognize that the difference is just projectional.

Focal Destructive Lesions

Osteomyelitis

- Hematogenous foci of infection tend to develop in the metaphyses of long bones.
- Usually there is at least a 7- to 10-day latent period between the onset of clinical symptoms and the first x-ray findings.

ACUTE

- Soft tissue swelling.
- Faint periosteal new bone formation — initially a subtle smudging of what should be a sharp, dense cortical line. A little later, a distinct layer of periosteal new bone develops.
- Slight focal demineralization progressing to patchy areas of trabecular bone loss.

CHRONIC

- Extensive bone destruction with irregular, sclerotic reaction.
- Sequestrum — dense, devascularized bone fragment lying within the pus and granulation tissue.
- Involucrum — peripheral shell of new supporting bone laid down by the periosteum.

The *radionuclide bone scan* plays a very significant role in the detection of bone infection. It is highly sensitive and shows a "hot spot" several days before any abnormalities become visible on x-ray film. In a child with clinical and laboratory features of infection, bone scan is indicated so that you can learn whether a bone focus is developing. It must be emphasized, however, that bone scans are etiologically nonspecific. A child who is limping, has a tender area on palpation and has a positive bone scan may have a tumor or a healing stress fracture rather than an infection. It is important also to be aware that scans will remain positive for long periods of time after the infection has been eradicated.

Tumors

A large variety of bone tumors exist. Most of them could be hypothesized on the basis of an assumption that any cell type normally found in bone could give origin to both benign and malignant tumors.[32] A sound grasp of this large topic is made possible, however, by the mastering of a few basic principles.

1. An x-ray showing an intraosseous lucency only informs you of the lack of normal bone structure; the lesion may be a fluid-filled cyst or may be composed of solid "water-density" tumor tissue such as cartilage, fibrous tissue or plasma cells.

2. Growth rate

● A benign, slowly growing lesion "e-x-p-a-n-d-s" bone and often has sharp, sclerotic margins.

● Primary bone malignancies infiltrate, permeate and violate anatomic boundaries.

3. There are predictable patterns based on radiographic appearance, patient age and site of bone involvement.

LESION	AGE	SITE	APPEARANCE
Simple cyst	Childhood	Metaphysis; central	Smooth, sharp, expansile
Benign cortical defect	Childhood	Metaphyseal cortex	Intracortical lucent defect with sclerotic margins
Giant cell tumor	20–40	Epiphysis	Well-demarcated, expansile destruction
Osteogenic sarcoma	5–20	Metaphysis	Mixed destruction and malignant bone formation with spicules radiating into soft tissues, periosteal bone reaction
Ewing's sarcoma	10–25	Diaphysis	Permeative medullary destruction with layered periosteal new bone

4. Bone metastases are usually multiple. Most are osteo-lytic; however, adenocarcinomas of the prostate and breast can evoke a "blastic" response, as can some forms of lymphoma. Primary bone tumors are very rare in middle-aged and elderly people; in such patients a destructive lesion, even a solitary one, is far more likely to be metastatic.

X-ray studies contribute in several ways to the diagnosis and management of bone tumor victims. The plain films disclose the lesion and show morphologic growth characteristics that permit, at the very least, a working hypothesis of benign versus malignant and, at times, a specific diagnosis. Benign cortical defects for instance, are radiologically pathognomonic and require no further attention. Simple cysts are quite characteristic. Although clinical management might require curettement and packing to prevent pathologic fracture, no preoperative staging workup or psychologic preparation is needed.

A malignant appearance obviously has very different implications. The plain films, sometimes with assistance by tomography, show a malignancy's growth characteristics and identify the most aggressive margin for the proper biopsy site. Angiography or computed tomography can more precisely define the boundaries of soft tissue extension so that the margins of the surgical resection can be planned. Chest films, liver

Fig 3–4.—Destructive bone lesions **A–C**. (Answer key on page 156.)

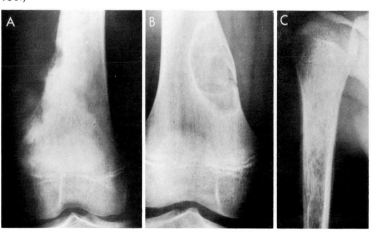

scans and bone scans are used in order to rule out distant metastases.

Three bone lesions are shown in Figure 3–4. Study them and decide whether they are neoplastic or inflammatory, benign or malignant, before checking the answers on page 156.

Metabolic Bone Disease

Adequate evaluation of diffuse metabolic bone disease requires a close correlation of x-ray, clinical and laboratory data. When therapeutic alternatives demand very precise differentiation among the diverse causes of osteopenia, sophisticated densitometric, isotopic and histochemical methods are available. Some generalities, however, are helpful in many clinical circumstances.

Osteoporosis

These "demineralized" bones have thin cortices and medullary trabeculae. Common etiologies include aging, disuse, Cushing's disease, osteogenesis imperfecta and hyperthyroidism. Many older women who present with a fracture of a vertebral body, proximal femur or distal radius have fractured through porotic bone.

Osteomalacia

This may look similar radiologically to osteoporosis but suspect it if:
- In an adult there are "pseudofractures" — seams of unmineralized osteoid along femoral necks, scapulae.
- In a child there are widened irregular growth plates (i.e., rickets).

Hyperparathyroidism

- Subperiosteal bone resorption — this early radiologic sign is best seen along the diaphyses of the phalanges, at the distal clavicles and along the lamina dura (tooth sockets).
- Diffuse demineralization.
- Focal lucent lesions — cysts and "brown tumors."

A significant percentage of patients with multiple myeloma present with *diffuse* demineralization only. They may later develop more focal destruction and ultimately show the widely recognized "punched-out" lesions.

In attempting to evaluate the adequacy of skeletal mineralization on standard x-rays, you should recognize that technical factors will exert enormous influence on the apparent density of the bones. A dark, densely exposed film will make bones look more lucent; an underexposed film leaves the bones more opaque. Use the soft tissue appearance as a clue to film penetration before trying to judge bone density.

Arthritis

The role of radiology:
- A supplement to your clinical and laboratory assessment of disease type.
- A followup tool to document progression of disease, suitability for surgical management or response to medical treatment.

A few "arthroradiologic" facts follow.[33]

Rheumatoid Arthritis

This is a systemic inflammatory disease with aggressive synovial proliferation causing destruction of cartilage, bone and supporting structures.

GROSS PATHOLOGY

Pannus, the invasive synovium, destroys cartilage and selectively erodes that portion (→) of intra-articular bone which is not protected by hyaline cartilage.

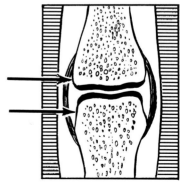

Fig 3–5. — Intra-articular anatomy.

Radiographic Findings

Early: slight demineralization, joint effusion, pericapsular swelling.

Mid: focal erosions along juxta-articular cortical margin, cartilage narrowing.

Late: massive destruction of bone and cartilage, subluxation, fibrous ankylosis.

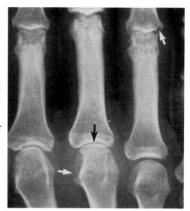

Fig 3–6. — Rheumatoid arthritis. Narrowed cartilage *(black arrow)*; marginal erosions *(white arrows)*.

Degenerative Arthritis

This is a noninflammatory deterioration of cartilage resulting in its flaking and fibrillation. Intra-articular irregularity, coupled with loss of cartilage elasticity and cushioning, leads to accelerated wear and reactive changes:

- narrowed cartilage
- reactive sclerosis of subchondral bone cortex
- osteophytic spurs along joint margins
- intraosseous subchondral cysts

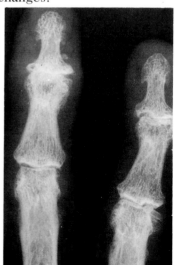

Fig 3–7. — Degenerative arthritis showing narrowing, sclerosis and osteophytes.

Gout

This disease of uric acid metabolism results in urate deposits within the joints and soft tissues.

INTRA-ARTICULAR

During an acute attack joint effusion may be visible. With repeated episodes, progressive gross destruction of the joint occurs.

TOPHI WITHIN THE SOFT TISSUES

These show as visible soft tissue nodularity, occasionally containing calcium. Cortical bone adjacent to a tophus becomes eroded, typically with sharp, sometimes overhanging margination.

LACK OF DEMINERALIZATION

This may be related to the intermittency of the attacks, permitting pain-free activity at other times.

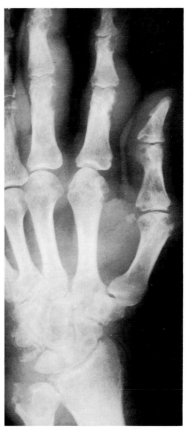

Fig 3–8.—Gout showing soft tissue tophi and multifocal bone destruction, often, but not always, at joints.

Septic Arthritis

This term refers to active bacterial infection of a joint. The pathogenesis is usually via hematogenous seeding or by extension from an adjacent osteomyelitis. You should note, however, that it may be iatrogenic, following aspiration of a sterile joint effusion or the administration of intra-articular medication.

RADIOGRAPHIC FINDINGS

- joint effusion, soft tissue swelling
- rapid cartilage and subchondral bone loss

Cartilage destruction is rapid and irreversible, requiring prompt diagnosis and treatment to avoid permanent joint damage. X-ray or clinical suspicion of this entity warrants immediate joint aspiration, smear and culture.

Ischemic Necrosis

This is not arthritis but can be mistaken for it clinically. Ischemia of the femoral head, coupled with the trauma of weight bearing, results in subcortical fissuring, fragmentation, sclerosis and collapse of the head. The articular cartilage is initially normal, as is the acetabular side of the joint, clues which immediately tell you this is not an arthritis.

There are several reasonable etiologies, such as femoral neck fractures, sickle cell anemia and caisson disease. Reasons for its occurrence in chronic pancreatitis and after prolonged steroid administration are more controversial.

In Figure 3–9, four painful joints are displayed. In each case the stage of disease is at least moderately advanced (early stages are not photogenic). List the diagnostic findings and conclusions for each before checking your answers on page 156.

The Spine

Although the vertebral column is subject to the same basic types of abnormalities as the extremities, the appearance of disease or injury here is modified by a more complicated anatomic structure. When you study spine radiographs, a basic format for analysis includes:

- orientation to projection and region
- study of adjacent soft tissues

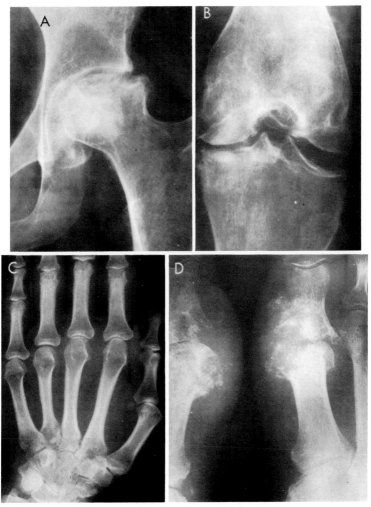

Fig 3–9.–Four painful joints **A–D**. (Answer key on page 156.)

- check of vertebral element alignment
- evaluation of disc space height
- assessment of overall mineralization
- search for lytic foci, linear fractures, compressions, anomalies

Satisfying yourself that all vertebral elements are present and intact is more challenging than looking for a hole in a long bone. Try the method used by Dr. Lucy Squire (Fig. 3–10).

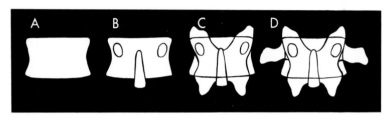

Fig 3–10.—Vertebral anatomy. **A,** body. **B,** add pedicles and spinous processes. **C,** plus lamina and facets. **D,** finish up with transverse processes.

Fig 3–11.—**A–C,** three patients with spine problems. **D** and **E,** a fourth patient, seen initially and again one year later. (Answer key on page 156.)

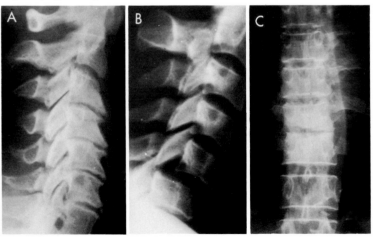

In Figure 3–11, four patients with serious vertebral abnormalities are shown. Trauma, infection, arthritis and neoplasm are represented. Attempt to describe and characterize the abnormalities before you check the answers on page 156.

SPECIAL PROCEDURES IN SKELETAL RADIOLOGY

PROCEDURE	APPLICATION
Tomography — delineation of a single body plane by a blurring out of other levels	Subtle fractures Small, obscured sequestrum in chronic osteomyelitis
Dynamic filming — plain films or cine recording of range of motion of a joint	Cervical subluxation in rheumatoid arthritis Temporomandibular joint mechanics in patients who "lock and click"
Stress views — films taken during judicious application of a deforming force	Suspected ligamentous tears of knee, ankle, acromioclavicular joint
Arthrography — intra-articular contrast material and air for study of a joint	Meniscus tears in the knee Glenohumeral capsular disruption
Arteriography — opacification and filming of regional arteries	Arterial injury in trauma Determination that a tumor is malignant by demonstration of a florid, disorganized vasculature
Radionuclide bone scan — scanning following administration of a radioactive isotope which is taken up by active bone	Earliest detector of metastatic disease to bone (when x-ray films are still negative)

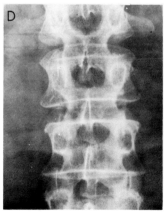 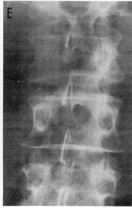

Fig 3–12.—A, asymmetric compression fracture L-1. **B,** tomography showing vertical fracture through lamina. **C,** rheumatoid arthritis, extension and flexion views show C1-2 instability *(arrows).* **D,** resting and stress views showing effects of medial collateral ligament injury.

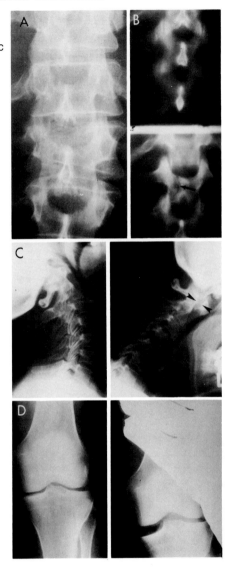

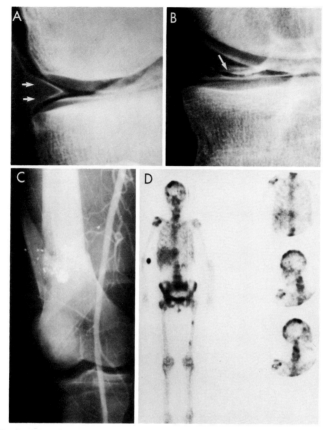

Fig 3–13.—**A,** cross-sectional profile of normal meniscus *(arrows)* on arthrography. **B,** meniscus tear *(arrow).* **C,** arteriogram following gunshot wound. Femoral artery is intact. **D,** metastatic foci showing as "hot spots" on radionuclide bone scan.

Special Studies

Additional x-ray studies of the skeletal system are frequently used in clinical problem solving when significant complaints or findings remain unclarified by basic filming (Fig 3–12, 3–13).

4

SPECIAL IMAGING TECHNIQUES

IN CHAPTER 5 we will study x-rays of the abdomen — plain film analysis and then the commonly utilized contrast studies of the digestive and urinary tracts. Those are the basic techniques for abdominal radiology, developed many decades ago and continuing to serve patients well.

Over the last 25 years angiography has emerged as a sophisticated tool for solving more complicated problems within the abdomen and retroperitoneum.[34] In the last five years, additional forms of diagnostic imaging have become available, providing accurate cross-sectional displays of internal structures with no effort, discomfort or risk for the patient.[35] These techniques are ultrasonography and computed tomography. They are marvelous tools for certain problems and absolutely useless for others.

In order to integrate remarks about angiography, ultrasound and computed tomography in later sections, it seems reasonable to stop at this point and consider their basic principles, strengths and limitations.

Angiography

Tremendous advances in angiographic capability have been achieved in the past decade. Many refined techniques are now available to help you care for your patients. *Rapid sequence* filming and cine studies offer assessment of functional as well as structural abnormality. Techniques using *steerable catheters* permit superselective catheterization of smaller branch arteries to yield better opacification and improved diagnostic detail. *Subtraction films* use photographic manipulation to remove overlying bone images from opacified vessels.

73

Geometric magnification, coupled with a small focal spot anode, improves the visualization of tiny blood vessels. A variety of *pharmacologic agents* is employed to improve vascular opacification and diagnostic accuracy.

Specific examinations are better considered within the context of each section of the manual, but some general concepts should be clarified now.

Terminology

"Angiography" is a general term describing any contrast study of the circulatory system. For purposes of clarity in your clinical communication, it is wise to be specific regarding the following terms:

Type of Vessel.—aortography, arteriography, angiocardiography, venography, lymphangiography. In the instance of "arteriograms," rapid sequence filming also provides images in the capillary and venous phases of that arterial distribution.

Body Part.—adrenal venogram, superior mesenteric arteriogram, pedal lymphangiogram, etc.

Applications of Vascular Catheterization

DELINEATION OF VESSELS

Intrinsic vascular disease.—Aneurysms, varices, vessel wall dissections, atherosclerotic plaques, lacerations, fistulas.

Extrinsic vessel displacement.—Adjacent space-occupying processes.

Neovascularity.—Delineation of vessels within malignant tumors and arteriovenous malformations.

VENOUS SAMPLING FOR BIOCHEMICAL ASSAY

Renal vein renin, adrenal vein corticosteroids, parathyroid vein parathormone.

THERAPEUTIC ANGIOGRAPHY

Vasoconstrictors in GI bleeding.
Embolization of tumors (Fig. 4–1), arteriovenous malforma-

Doppler instruments utilize ultrasound frequency shifts to detect and quantitate flood flow.

"B-scanning" is the display mode used for anatomic imaging of abdominal structures. The ultrasonic transducer is attached to a jointed, mechanical arm which is equipped with positional and angle sensing devices. The probe is moved back and forth along a body contour; echo signals are built up on a storage type oscilloscope, and a sectional view of the region is obtained. Transverse and sagittal sections are made, initially at 2 cm intervals. However, as areas of concern begin to emerge, intervening or obliquely oriented planes can be supplemented. Photographs taken of the display tube then provide a permanent record of the images (Fig 4–2).

Ultrasonic imaging is well suited to mapping out organs, major vessels and pathologic masses, showing their outlines but also providing information about their internal architecture. Waves transmitted through cysts encounter no reflective interfaces other than their walls, resulting in a "sonolucent" or "anechoic" appearance. Solid structures generally show internal echoes, although there are exceptions.

Ultrasound, in the physical ranges used in medical imaging,

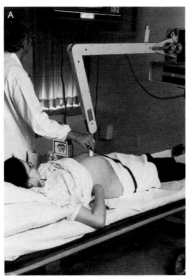
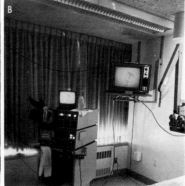

Fig 4–2. — Ultrasound examining room. **A,** obstetrical study in progress. **B,** ultrasound unit and monitoring device.

cannot "see" behind bone. Obviously that poses problems high in the upper abdomen where the rib cage attempts to shield such structures as the adrenals and upper poles of kidneys. Creative approaches to scanning with angulated beams or along intercostal spaces constitute some of the "art" of ultrasound. Barium within the GI tract is also a barrier to ultrasound transmission and will prevent satisfactory study.

Ultrasound is badly deflected by gas-containing structures. It cannot be used for imaging through intervening lung, and for this reason chest applications are limited to the heart, the great vessels and pleura. Unfortunately intervening bowel gas can interfere substantially with supine abdominal imaging in some patients. Liver and gallbladder images, however, are usually cephalad to the major gas collections, while renal and retroperitoneal imaging can be well accomplished from a posterior approach.

Computed Tomography

Computed tomography (CT) was developed in Great Britain and then was introduced into the United States in 1973. Initial installations were entirely for intracranial imaging. By 1975 body units were in operation, and preliminary reports on their usefulness began appearing in the literature.

CT is an x-ray method of producing a cross-sectional body image that depicts extremely subtle differences in tissue density. The image is not really an x-ray picture but rather a mathematical reconstruction based on many thousands of density measurements of tiny tissue volumes. Tissue attenuation differences as small as 0.5% are detectable, making it possible, in intracranial work for instance, to differentiate white matter, gray matter, ventricular cerebrospinal fluid, edema, hemorrhage and tumor. All of these would formerly have been perceived as "soft tissue densities" and have been differentiable only by means of arteriography or pneumoencephalography. The sensitivity of CT can be increased under some circumstances by concurrent administration of an intravenous iodinated contrast agent.

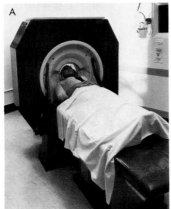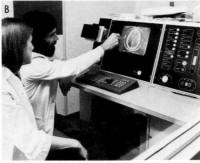

Fig 4–3. — Computed tomography suite. **A,** patient positioned in head unit. **B,** console.

CT units differ in many details but have fundamental components in common. Figure 4–3 shows the essential elements: patient stretcher, circular gantry housing the x-ray tube and detector systems, computer manipulation and data storage units and viewing and recording console. Within the gantry, the tube/detector system traverses the body part, rotates a few degrees, repeats the traverse, rotates again and repeats this process for a complete 180 degrees coverage. The patient is then shifted, perhaps 2 cm depending on the body part under study, and the next "slice" is made.

These installations are expensive, costing from one-half to three-quarters of a million dollars each, and have high maintenance and operational costs. Consequently, examinations are expensive, in the range of $250 to $300. Do these examinations simply add to the patient's diagnostic burden, or do they substitute for other expensive, higher risk examinations? Radiologists at Mallinckrodt Institute in St. Louis have documented a "66%, 34% and 29% reduction in pneumoencephalograms, cerebral angiograms, and radionuclide brain scans respectively, since installation of CT head scanning equipment."[13] Parallel data on body scanning is now accumulating and is being watched very carefully by physicians, consumers and health care planners.[14] Initially, in order to develop valid data comparing the accuracy of CT, ultrasound, radionuclide scans and angiography, there will be a stage during which redundant, overlapping imaging techniques will have to be employed.

Your medical training is occurring during this exploratory, transitional stage. You will be participating in selections, seeing results, forming your own conclusions and studying the accumulated data of others. Enjoy the excitement of this period but guard against developing long-term habits of ordering everything for everyone.

If it becomes solidly established that CT and ultrasound are equally good for one particular problem, CT should be dropped in favor of the less expensive examination. It may emerge that CT can provide unique information about the extent of an intra-abdominal mass but that angiography is also needed preoperatively to accurately map out vascular connections for the surgeon.

The indications and interactions of available diagnostic technology will continue to require your attention over the years as you attempt to provide quality care for your patients.

5

ABDOMINAL FILMS

WHEN THE INTRINSIC DIAGNOSTIC POTENTIALS of plain abdominal and thoracic films are compared, we note some basic disadvantages below the diaphragm. The major one is that the superb natural contrast of air is less generously available, normally limited to the gastrointestinal tract and then present only in undependable quantities and distributions. Despite this, a knowledge of anatomy, familiarity with the known manifestations of common diseases and a willingness to pursue suspicions by sensible application of special studies will enable a physician to achieve a high degree of diagnostic specificity.[36]

Problems in Terminology

Before plunging into the details of radiologic data collection, consider a frequently voiced question: "How do I word my request for an abdominal x-ray?" In the chest and extremities, frontal and lateral projections are almost always a good starting point. Depending on what they show, the need for additional views may become apparent. In the abdomen, standard routines too often overfilm some problems and fall short in others. It therefore makes more sense to tailor the initial examination to your patient's needs. For example:

- An AP supine film of the abdomen will be all that you need to show renal size, a lost surgical sponge, an ingested foreign body or most forms of calcification and calculi. Calcifications of the pancreatic head and those within aortic aneurysms may overlie the spine, however. If the history or physical examination makes you suspect these conditions, request a lateral view in addition to the AP.

81

- When your concern is obstruction or perforation, be sure to request upright or lateral decubitus films in addition to the AP supine. This will be discussed later in more detail.
- A baby with anal atresia is sometimes filmed upside down with a lead marker taped to his anal dimple to show its distance from the distal rectal gas bubble.

Do not let yourself get confused by the terminology.

Urologists say "KUB" — they are primarily interested in Kidneys, Ureters and Bladder.

Radiologists say plain or scout film — we are eager to proceed to a contrast study.

Anachronists say "flat plate" — fondly recalling the days when plate glass rather than plastic base carried the photosensitive silver emulsion.

"AP abdomen" best parallels other standard terminology such as PA chest and lateral skull. By convention that *will* be supine unless you request an upright projection.

Study Method

Do not just gaze *at* the film; look *for* specific things, and make a conscious effort to detect or exclude them.

Technical Check

Ascertain the adequacy of filming technique and make a conscious notation of the patient's position and of the radiographic projection. Those in common usage include AP supine, oblique, lateral, lateral decubitus and upright. Only the last two are made with a horizontal beam and can show air-fluid levels in the bowel or detect free intraperitoneal air.

Survey of the "Unrelated"

- Lung bases. Basilar pneumonia or pleuritis can mimic abdominal disease clinically.
- Extra-abdominal soft tissues. An incarcerated hernia may be the cause of your patient's bowel obstruction.

● Skeletal structures. Check the ribs, pelvis and lumbar spine. Fractures, destructive foci or congenital anomalies might relate directly to the abdominal problem but would, in any event, have clinical significance for the patient.

Fat and Muscle Planes

Identify the margins of the psoas muscles and the linear radiolucent flank stripes (Fig 5–1).

These are obscured by processes that infiltrate the fat with water-density material—pus, blood, tumor.

EXAMPLE: loss of lower right flank stripe in appendiceal abscess.

Fig 5–1.—Normal supine AP abdomen.

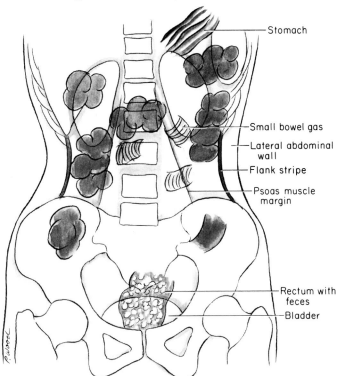

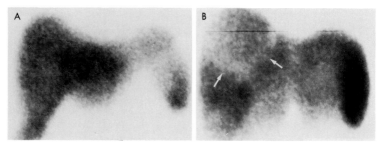

Fig 5–2. — Liver-spleen radionuclide scan. **A,** normal. **B,** large abscess superior portion right lobe *(arrows)*.

Solid Organs

Identify the liver, spleen, kidneys — checking for size, position, margins and homogeneity.

The plain film evaluation of spleen and liver size is only a gross assessment. It should be appreciated also that the lower liver margin seen on an abdominal film is often the posterior one and may not correspond to the palpable anterior edge. Radionuclide liver and spleen scans can provide you with more precise volume determinations, as well as information regarding their internal structure (Fig 5–2). Renal size, shape and position are very often easily seen on good quality films.

Computed tomography provides useful images of solid abdominal and retroperitoneal structures along with the tissues which surround them (Fig 5–3).

Gas Pattern

Is anything displaced or distended?

Sizable quantities of air can be expected normally in stomach and colon. The presence of gas within the small bowel, especially in hospitalized patients, is *not* abnormal if the bowel is not actually dilated. This condition, the result of air swallowing, is frequently seen in patients with dyspnea, pain or anxiety. When looking at the "scout" or preliminary film for a contrast study, remember that laxatives or enemas have been administered and that sometimes a "purged gut gathers gas."

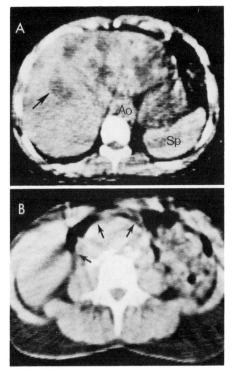

Fig 5–3. — Computed tomography of abdomen. **A,** multiple hepatic cysts; largest indicated by *arrow.* **B,** retroperitoneal adenopathy *(arrows).*

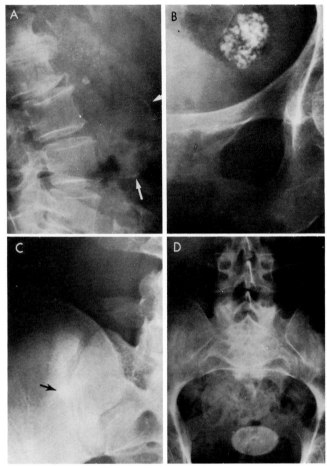

Fig 5–4. — Abdominal calcifications. **A,** aortic aneurysm *(arrows).* **B,** uterine fibroid. This was an incidental finding in woman with breast cancer metastases to left ischium. **C,** appendiceal fecalith *(arrow).* **D,** bladder calculus.

Calcifications

Common but often unimportant:
    costal cartilages
    phleboliths in pelvic venous plexus
    atherosclerotic plaques
    old granulomas in nodes, spleen
    calcified uterine fibroids
Common and very important (Fig 5–4):
    biliary calculi
    urinary calculi
    pancreatic calcifications
    aneurysms
    appendiceal fecaliths

Intraperitoneal Air and Fluid

These are important, often catastrophic, findings which must be recognized! They will be discussed in detail later in the chapter.

To summarize your study routine then, you began by checking the bones, soft tissues, solid organs and gas pattern. You then completed your search by looking for calcifications, ascites and free air.

Portable Films of the Abdomen
(An exercise in futility)

The overall tissue density of the abdomen is far greater than that of the chest; considerably more radiation is required for adequate exposure. In many hospitals today, the portable x-ray unit can achieve adequate exposure only by increasing the exposure time. During the prolonged interval required in normally nourished adults, breathing, involuntary motion and peristalsis will frequently degrade the image.

If clinically important information is being sought, your patient should be filmed in the x-ray department. If he is seriously ill, accompany him down at a prearranged moment when he can be studied promptly and then returned as soon as the film is checked. With rapid automatic processing, the film-checking delay is insignificant and may save him another trip if the film shows something that requires clarification on another view.

Dilated Bowel

Basic Rules and Classic Patterns

PARALYTIC ILEUS

Findings
- Peristalsis has stopped, and there is now diffuse distension of *small* and *large bowel* (Fig 5–5) by gas and fluid. Filming in the upright position shows balanced air-fluid levels in long slack loops.

Causes
- Peritonitis, trauma, drug effect and bowel ischemia.

MECHANICAL OBSTRUCTION

Findings
- Proximal to the lesion, the gut is distended with gas and fluid in a "stepladder" distribution; distally the gut is empty (Fig 5–6, A).
- Upright films (Fig 5–6, B) show air-fluid levels with tight, "hairpin" loops.

Causes
- In the adult consider adhesions, hernia, tumor, intussusception, volvulus and gallstone ileus.
- In infants consider the distended stomach of pyloric stenosis, the "double bubble" of duodenal atresia, and small bowel obstructions due to ileal atresia and meconium ileus.

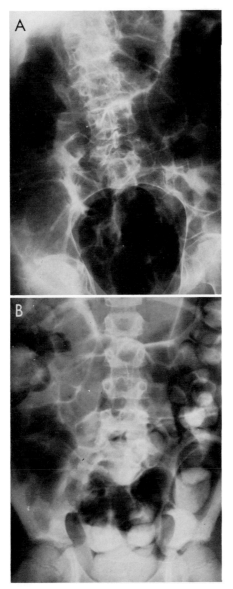

Fig 5–5.—Dilated bowel. **A,** paralytic ileus showing dilatation of colon and small bowel. **B,** fecal impaction.

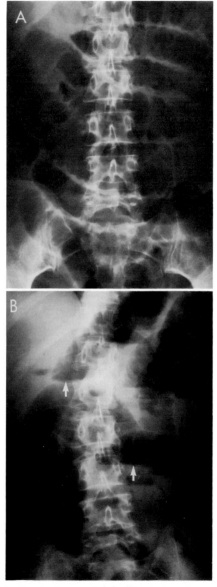

Fig 5–6.—Mechanical small bowel obstruction. **A,** supine. **B,** upright, showing air-fluid levels.

Modifications (and Annoying Exceptions)

PARTIAL OR VERY RECENT OBSTRUCTION

Distal emptying may be as yet incomplete and radiologic findings initially inconclusive. Follow-up films, clinical correlation or contrast studies will clarify the issue.

THE "ENEMA ARTIFACT"

Distal to a small bowel obstruction, a pathologically emptied colon can be factitiously refilled by a well-intentioned but poorly timed cleansing enema. If that enema was administered before the films were made, you could be badly misled.

SENTINEL LOOP SIGN

Localized paralysis and dilatation of a bowel segment may occur adjacent to an area of intense inflammation. This can be seen with acute appendicitis, cholecystitis and pancreatitis.

MESENTERIC THROMBOSIS

Mesenteric thrombosic can mimic anything. You should be highly suspicious, however, if:
- Bowel dilatation is in the anatomic distribution of the superior mesenteric artery.
- Bowel wall edema is present, causing nodular or "thumbprinting" configurations of the intestinal gas shadows.

The late stages of bowel infarction may show linear streaks of gas within the wall of necrotic bowel and branching patterns of gas within the intrahepatic radicals of the portal vein.

Supplementary Procedures in Suspected Obstruction

If the diagnosis remains uncertain after plain films and clinical findings are closely correlated but a decision must be made regarding possible surgical intervention, a more definitive procedure must be selected. Ultrasound, computed tomography and angiography do not have useful roles here. Opacification of the gastrointestinal tract is what is required. The questions are via what route and with what agents?

COLONIC OBSTRUCTION SUSPECTED OR POSSIBLE

- We would do a barium enema and outline the lesion from below. Barium in the colon *proximal* to an obstruction can desiccate, harden and contribute to further obstruction. Barium *distal* to an obstruction will be promptly evacuated.

COLONIC OBSTRUCTION ABSENT

The plain films show small bowel dilatation but are equivocal in differentiating paralytic ileus from mechanical small bowel obstruction.

- We would need to study your patient from above. The choice of contrast agents, however, is controversial.

Barium will give a denser, more definitive image for better delineation of the site and the nature of the lesion. If the patient goes on to surgery, there may be a time in the early postoperative period when peristalsis is very sluggish. Large residual amounts of barium remaining in the colon could contribute to constipation.

An iodinated, water-soluble agent will be propelled rapidly toward the ileocecal valve but will be diluted by the intraluminal fluid and give a hazier end-point. While the agent would not contribute to postoperative obstipation, there is a more immediate potential danger in its use. It is very hypertonic, will draw fluid into the bowel and can cause hypovolemia. This could pose a particular threat in infants and children; surveillance over intravascular fluid volumes must be maintained.

Intraperitoneal Air

Perforations of peptic ulcers and colonic diverticula are the catastrophic events generally responsible for intraperitoneal air. Because of an intense inflammatory response, appendiceal perforation will more often result in a walled-off abscess, sometimes containing tiny bacterogenic gas bubbles. Free intraperitoneal air may be an innocuous finding for several days following abdominal surgery, tubal insufflation or peritoneal dialysis.

Plain Films

The details of patient transport and filming sequence are important and demand close coordination among clinician, technician and radiologist.[15] At the close of the physical examination, your patient is supine, and his intraperitoneal gas is spread out in little bubbles under his anterior abdominal wall. We need to make those bubbles coalesce and migrate to an area where we can see them. If he comes supine to the x-ray department and we prop him up and promptly take a film, the gas may not have had a chance to migrate up to a visible, subdiaphragmatic location. The patient then will suffer the consequences of a missed or delayed diagnosis.

Because such a patient is often too ill to be transported upright, develop the policy of sending him to us lying on his *left* side. Our first film should be a horizontal beam view of his right side, in which intraperitoneal air will be visible between his liver and his thoracoabdominal wall. This *left lateral decubitus* film, then, is deliberately arranged after he has been in that position for 10 minutes. Without permitting resumption of the supine position, we can then sit him upright and get frontal and lateral chest films. If the patient can tolerate it, the upright chest film is a fine way to detect a thin crescentic radiolucency beneath the diaphragm. "Upright abdomen," of the sort we employ looking for air-fluid levels in bowel loops, has the central ray aimed at the navel and does not hit the diaphragm tangentially. To complete the examination we then obtain a supine film.

The sequence: 1. "staged" left lateral decubitus abdomen
2. upright chest — frontal and lateral
3. supine abdomen

Contrast Studies

If asked to localize the precise site of perforation, we will use iodinated water-soluble material. Nothing is totally innocuous in the peritoneal cavity, but this is probably better than barium.

If we cannot detect the perforation but a followup film a few minutes later shows a dense urogram, the leak has not sealed off. The organic iodine in these contrast materials is poorly absorbed by the intact gut but will be well absorbed by the peritoneal surface.

Ascites

The overall "ground-glass" appearance that is popularly advertised for ascites can be faked by obesity or by a light, underpenetrated filming technique. Ascites of that magnitude is clinically obvious. However, smaller, clinically inapparent quantities can often be demonstrated on supine abdominal films.

Progressive Accumulation—Supine Position

- The first few hundred cc's pool in the posterior hollow of the pelvis, showing as a rounded, water-density "mass" superior to the bladder and overlying the sacrum (Fig 5–7, A, B).
- As the volume increases, fluid begins to extend superolaterally out of the pelvis. At this stage the appearance has been likened to "dog ears" (Fig 5–7, C). Loops of small bowel normally occupy portions of the true pelvis. If they contain fluid they will mimic this "dog ear" configuration. Ultrasound could sort this out, if it were a significant issue.
- When the total reaches about 500 cc, fluid runs up along the lateral gutters, displacing the colon medially from the radiolucent flank stripes (Fig 5–7, D).
- With increasing volumes, the inferior margins of the spleen and liver float away from adjacent fat, and their profiles are lost.

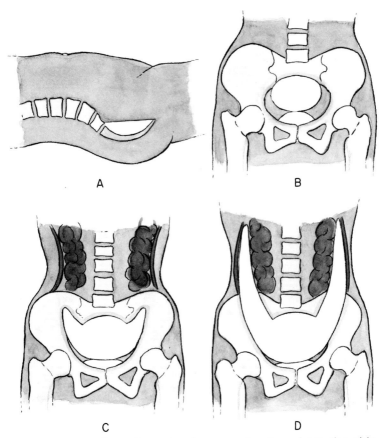

Fig 5–7. – Ascites. **A,** anatomic reconstruction, from the side.
B, C, D, sketches of supine radiography showing increasing volumes
of ascitic fluid.

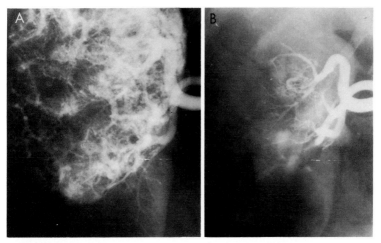

Fig 4–1.—Highly vascular renal malignancy before **(A)** and after **(B)** embolization with Gelfoam fragments. Note massive occlusions of intrarenal vessels. Procedure was done immediately before nephrectomy.

tions, esophageal varices, etc. Embolic materials being used include clot, Gelfoam, plastic beads, steel coils, and polymerizing tissue adhesives.

Ultrasonography

Echo devices are based on the sonar principle of determining distance by measuring round-trip transit time of a high frequency sound wave. In a probe or transducer, an electrical impulse is converted to a mechanical compressive pulse which is transmitted to the patient's surface. The wave traverses body tissues and is reflected from acoustical interfaces, returning to the receiver portion of the transducer.[12]

Several types of display formats are available, each well suited for specific types of diagnostic imaging. "A" mode displays show echo amplitudes and depths on an oscilloscope and can be used to determine whether the midline structures of the brain are shifted. "T-M" mode displays are suited to investigation of pulsatile structures as in echocardiography.

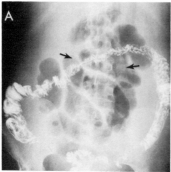

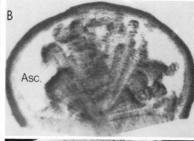

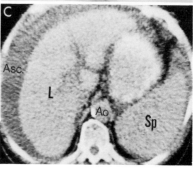

Fig 5–8. — Ascites. **A,** supine films made at termination of barium enema. Colonic position is fixed, but small bowel floats centrally. Note preserved psoas margin *(arrows).* **B,** transverse ultrasound section at level of umbilicus. Echo-free fluid is visible laterally in flanks. **C,** computed tomogram high in abdomen. Ascitic fluid (Asc) of low attenuation coefficient lies lateral to liver (L). Ao-aorta, Sp-spleen.

- Finally, as the abdomen becomes distended with fluid, bowel loops float centrally but remain separated from one another (Fig 5–8).

Abdominal Trauma

Clinical Considerations

Emergency room evaluation and initial handling of badly injured patients may need to include airway management, stabilization of blood volume and splinting of fractures. These measures should be taken *before* the patient is transported to the x-ray department. The clinician should also be aware of the potential for sudden deterioration in the patient's condition. Radiology departments have developed special techniques for handling and filming acutely injured people. However, the concerned clinician accompanies this type of patient to the department to guide us in moving injured parts and to maintain surveillance over the patient's systemic status.

Radiologic Considerations

Depending on the type and extent of injury, various combinations of findings may be evident on plain films of the abdomen:

- fractures
- obliteration of normal fat planes and visceral margins
- peritoneal fluid (blood)
- peritoneal air

The presence of hematuria dictates the need for radiologic exploration of the urinary tract. This begins with excretory urography but retrograde cystography may also be required if pelvic injury is suspected. Emergency arteriography and radioisotope scans can provide definitive information in suspected lacerations of solid organs. The extent of the radiologic assessment obviously will depend on the clinical circumstances. In suspected multiorgan injuries, the surgeon needs all the preoperative angiographic information possible because some areas are difficult to see adequately and others require a much more prolonged exploration. However, in a persistently hemorrhaging patient, with rapidly deteriorating vital signs, immediate surgery without preoperative angiography is often necessary.

Abdominal Masses

Certain types of abdominal and retroperitoneal masses are more logically discussed within the chapters on digestive, urinary and reproductive systems. Often, however, a patient comes to you because he "feels something," or you palpate an unsuspected mass on routine physical examination. Unless there are other clinical features to steer you to a particular organ system, the next step requires some thought.

One approach would be to opacify everything that has a

lumen and send us one untidy requisition asking for an upper GI, small bowel, barium enema, oral cholecystogram, and excretory urogram. In your pocket for later you keep another requisition asking for an aortogram, lymphangiogram, vena cavagram and hysterosalpingogram. I am obviously joking, but also reminding you of the number of structures we *can* "light up" for you. Capability, of course, is no reason for an examination, so let us try a little different approach.

An exploratory laparotomy would be the fastest way to find out what was in there. If the mass was an ovarian dermoid or a benign mesenteric cyst, its resection would be straightforward, and you could take pride in having reached a rapid, relatively inexpensive solution. On the other hand, you may not

Fig 5–9.—Longitudinal ultrasound scans of abdominal masses. **A,** pancreatic pseudocyst. Large sonolucent mass connecting *(arrow)* to smaller one posteriorly. **B,** aortic aneurysm with clot and plaque *(arrow)* posteriorly.

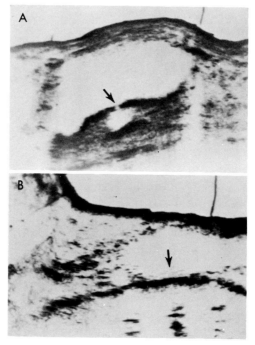

have been ready to take on an aortic aneurysm; a renal cyst should have been managed by percutaneous puncture, and an intra-abdominal malignancy should have been "staged" for proper management.

A rational, directed workup might start with an ultrasound examination to find out whether the mass is cystic or solid and to determine whether it is arising from an organ or from adjacent tissues. An aortic aneurysm, a pancreatic pseudocyst (Fig 5–9) or an intrarenal lesion may be definitively outlined in that manner. A computed tomography scan might offer better anatomic information if a high posterior mass needs to be localized to determine whether it is of renal, adrenal or posterior hepatic origin. Findings on one of these screening examinations would then determine the direction of further workup; a long list of available procedures doomed to be irrelevant would be bypassed.

6

GASTROINTESTINAL EXAMINATIONS

THE LIMITATIONS of plain abdominal films in gastrointestinal problem solving are obvious. Ever since Cannon fed bismuth to a cat in 1897, we have searched for better ways to look at living gut. Radiologic examinations provide one parameter in gastrointestinal diagnosis. In some instances the radiographic appearance and fluoroscopic behavior of a lesion are absolutely diagnostic.[37] In other situations the x-ray findings are equivocal or serve only to corroborate impressions gleaned from endoscopy, manometry or absorption studies. The various clinical and radiologic investigations complement rather than compete with each other. Thoughtful selection and integration are required.

Preparation for Barium Examination

Bowel Preps

When one studies a hollow tube radiologically, the configuration of its lumen and the appearance of its mucosal surface can be well assessed only when it is empty. For *upper gastrointestinal* (UGI) work, it is ordinarily sufficient that the patient has taken nothing by mouth since the previous evening. If your patient's history, however, suggests that pyloric scarring may be producing gastric outlet obstruction, a nasogastric tube should be passed and his stomach emptied before the examination. Otherwise barium will drift, settle, flocculate, dilute out and do everything *but* outline the problem.

Achieving a clean colon for *barium enema* study is more difficult. The details of preparation vary widely. You will find

101

that your consultant radiologist has developed a detailed instruction list for outpatients and for the nursing staff to use with inpatients. Most good preparations include a 2-day liquid diet, a moderately powerful cathartic the evening before and an early morning suppository. Some radiologists feel that cleansing enemas are necessary, while others believe that these leave colons fluid-filled and irritable. An "average" cathartic dose will absolutely "wring out" some patients and produce feeble cramping but no results in others. Consult with your radiologist regarding individualized modifications for patients with conditions such as active colitis or profound constipation. With hospitalization costs so staggering, you may be tempted to try to cut corners and abbreviate bowel preps. This is often unsuccessful. After futile attempts to distinguish adherent feces from polyps, the radiologist may have to report this to you as a compromised, substandard examination, one that requires repetition after re-preparation. Barium examinations are readily performed on outpatients, but if you do plan to hospitalize your patient for overall diagnosis and management, x-ray examination can be prescheduled and bowel preparation begun at home.

People Preps

Preparing your patient psychologically is as important as cleansing his intestine. Every effort should be made to help him to understand why the examination is being done, what it will be like and how the results will be made known to him. The first two issues are important but self-explanatory, although I should remind you that if *you* have never seen the procedure, you will not be able to describe it accurately or in a helpful way.

The third issue merits further exploration. At the close of the examination, the radiologist will often know something important, possibly even grim, about the patient's illness. He does not, however, possess the full clinical data; he knows nothing of your patient's emotional stability or maturity and should not be the one to convey the results. Your patient should be made aware of this policy, lest he misinterpret the radiologist's noncommittal farewell as detached, discourteous or even ominous.

Out of consideration for the other waiting, starving patients, the fluoroscopist will often move along pretty briskly. After greeting the patient and introducing himself he will probably ask a few questions and amplify some of the relevant symptomatology but will not usually encourage prolonged discourse on tangential subjects. Once the examination is under way, concentration on what he is doing and seeing will probably limit his conversation to requests for swallowing, breathing and positioning. His parting comments will be courteous but not especially informative. Some radiologists will be able to convey warmth and concern during this brief, two-dimensional encounter; others will not. An occasional patient whom you have not prepared well for the experience will come away with a feeling that the examination was a "dehumanizing" experience. It really need not be.

The Procedures

The Upper GI Series

Following a scout film of the abdomen, the patient drinks a flavored barium sulfate suspension and is fluoroscoped and positioned as the opaque bolus of barium and air is followed. Barium is heavy; air is light. Some structures are anterior and others posterior. Patients are made to assume upright, prone, supine and oblique positions. These are the controllable conditions that permit us to distend, empty and coat each segment of esophagus, stomach and duodenum in a few minutes of intermittent fluoroscopy.

Portions of this spectacle are permanently recorded on small spot films, cine recording or video tapes, the radiologist's judgment determining the details of this selection. He is no more likely to record an entire examination on tape than a surgeon would routinely document every abdominal exploration with movies.

Following completion of fluoroscopy and spot filming, the radiologist selects certain views to be taken subsequently by the technician on full-sized x-ray films.

The Small Bowel Examination

The traditional UGI series ends at the ligament of Treitz. We will study the gut from there to the cecum when your request or the patient's comments alert us to the possibility of small bowel disease. At the completion of the UGI, the patient will be given additional barium to drink, and sequential abdominal films will be taken, perhaps at 20- to 30-minute intervals. Between films the patient is returned to a waiting area and the fluoroscopist goes on to examine other patients. He is shown each interval film, however, and at any point may bring the patient back in for further fluoroscopy and spot filming. "Running the small bowel" may take anywhere from 30 minutes to 5 hours or more depending on its intrinsic transit time. The additional effort, expense and radiation are all reasons why the "small bowel follow-through" should not be part of a routine GI examination. If selected and performed for reasonable indications, it has a good diagnostic yield in neoplastic, inflammatory and certain malabsorptive diseases.

The Barium Enema

The abdominal scout film is viewed, and if no substantial amount of colonic feces is detected, a catheter is inserted into the patient's rectum. Ordinarily one with a slightly bulbous plastic tip is used. If the patient is elderly, debilitated or has had problems "holding" enemas before, a soft, inflatable bulb retention catheter will be selected. Under fluoroscopic control the opaque enema is administered, while retrograde fill of the colon is closely observed and spot filmed back to the distal ileum. Large "filled" films are obtained in a variety of projections, followed by a "postevacuation" film to show coated mucosa and empty bowel. Air may then be introduced, providing an air-distended, barium coated mucosal image. This is the air-contrast examination, a sensitive detector of small polyps.

Most patients do not recall their barium enemas with any great enthusiasm, and an occasional individual will be relatively uncomfortable during it. The majority report their perceptions as ranging from distaste to mild discomfort.

Modifications of Barium Studies for Special Problems

● Cine or video tape recording to capture subtle or transitory findings — motility problems, esophageal webs, tiny tracheoesophageal fistulae. These recordings can be replayed and meticulously analyzed by a group of consultants long after the patient has returned to his room.
● Mechanical maneuvers to demonstrate gastroesophageal reflux — straining, prone Trendelenburg position, abdominal compression.
● Breathing maneuvers to alter intrathoracic pressure and venous distention while esophageal varices are sought.
● Use of pharmacologic enhancement:
1. Glucagon is employed in selected circumstances to cause transient paralysis of peristalsis. In hypotonic duodenography, the duodenal loop is paralyzed so that its medial wall can be studied for subtle effects by an abnormal pancreas. Glucagon is also used when a barium enema shows segmental narrowing and the diagnostic question is spasm versus constricting lesion.
2. Neostigmine (a cholinergic stimulant) is occasionally used to increase intestinal motility for a more convenient study of the small bowel. Those 5-hour transit times are hard on everybody, especially the patient.

Interpretation

Quick Review of Normal Data

Contemplate your baseline of normal facts regarding each segment of gut from pharynx to rectum: anatomic location, shape, caliber, mucosal characteristics.

Film Display

Put up the large films first for easy recognition, and then "spots" as you get them oriented.

Functional Assessment

If at this moment the radiologist or his report is not present, you are at a serious disadvantage. The GI tract is a shifting, churning, writhing thing, but this activity is orderly and purposeful when viewed fluoroscopically. The spot films, however, capture one moment in time, a moment when peristaltic waves may look like strictures and transiently trapped barium mimics ulcerations. The importance of the fluoroscopic information should never be underestimated.

Examples of some entities that are evident fluoroscopically but cannot be detected on films alone are: esophageal scleroderma, gastroesophageal reflux, infiltrated gastric wall, irritable duodenal bulb.

Morphologic Assessment

Remember, we are just stuffing lumens and coating linings; only indirectly do we get information about mural and serosal characteristics. For instance, we speak of excess barium collections as pockets, flecks and niches and realize that they are outlining ulcers and diverticula. "Filling defects" are relative lucencies within the barium column caused by protruding tissue or intraluminal objects such as masses, foreign bodies and feces.

GI TRACT LESIONS

The sketches in Figure 6–1 could be modified to portray any segment of the GI tract.[1] As a matter of fact, because a limited number of things can happen to any hollow tube, similar deformities could befall the ureters, blood vessels, bronchi and spinal subarachnoid space. Figure 6–2 illustrates some specific GI abnormalities encountered with great frequency in clinical practice.

The Acute GI Bleeder

The patient with acute, massive GI bleeding requires a very different approach to diagnosis and management. It is not

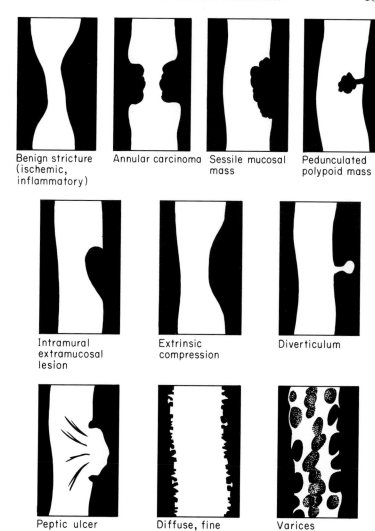

Fig 6–1.—GI tract lesions; sketches of classical configurations (after Squire[1]).

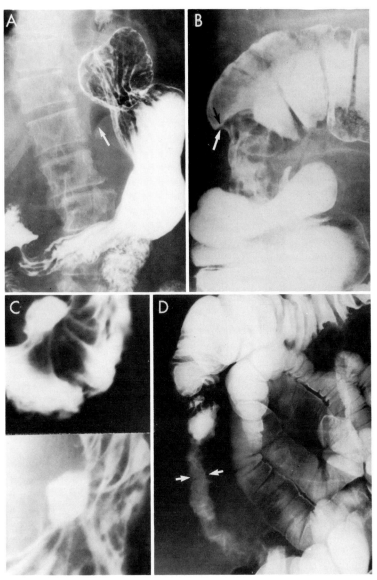

Fig 6–2.—Common GI lesions. **A,** hiatus hernia. *Arrow* shows level of diaphragm. **B,** annular carcinoma of ascending colon. Note overhanging edges *(arrows)*. **C,** benign gastric ulcer on fluoroscopic spot films. **D,** regional enteritis. Terminal ileum is thick, nodular and irregular *(arrows)*.

simply a question of doing the same things, only faster. Barium studies will interfere with other more promising examinations, and are very likely to be unsuccessful for several reasons:

- The patient is virtually immobilized by blood pressure cuffs and transfusion IVs and cannot be turned and positioned optimally.
- Detection of ulcers and neoplasms requires an empty stomach and the opportunity for barium to smoothly coat the mucosal folds. Retained secretions and floating blood clots will subvert adequate examination.
- The eroded areas in acute hemorrhagic gastritis are extremely superficial, do not accumulate barium and are rarely diagnosed radiologically.

Stabilize the patient's vital signs, lavage his stomach and ponder the relative merits of endoscopy and arteriography. Your clinical suspicions regarding the etiology of the bleeding and the local availability of endoscopic and angiographic consultants will influence your choice.

Arteriography in GI Problems

Transfemoral catheterization of the aorta provides access to the mesenteric arteries as well as to major branches of the celiac axis. Circulatory structure and function of all of the gut from gastric cardia to distal colon can therefore be examined as rapid sequential filming outlines the arterial, capillary and portal venous phases.

GI Bleeding

During active bleeding (1 – 2 cc/minute), contrast material may appear within the bowel lumen following intra-arterial injection. The catheter can then be left in place and used for perfusion with a vasoconstrictor (Fig 6 – 3).

Occasionally a patient is plagued by episodic GI bleeding from a site not disclosed by repeated conventional barium or endoscopic studies. Lesions such as hemangiomas, angiodysplasias and subtle neoplasms may be responsible. These are often detectable angiographically.

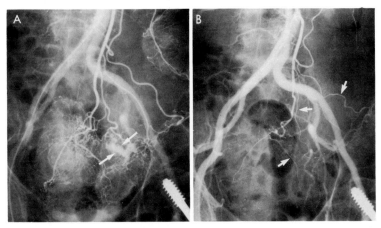

Fig 6–3.—Massive hemorrhage from colonic diverticulum. **A,** inferior mesenteric arteriogram showing contrast extravasating into bowel lumen *(arrows)*. **B,** bleeding stopped by intra-arterial Pitressin infusion. Note constriction of branches *(arrows)* of inferior mesenteric artery compared to preinfusion appearance. (History of previous left hip fracture and pinning).

Ischemic Disease

In patients with mesenteric angina, arteriography may delineate proximal arterial lesions amenable to surgical correction.

Portal Hypertension

Several routes of access are available for study of the portal circulation to delineate occlusions and collateral circulation. For those patients with portal hypertension in whom surgical management is under consideration, preoperative evaluation is critical. A technique is now emerging for transhepatic catheterization of the portal vein and its branches to permit therapeutic embolization of esophageal varices.

Intra-abdominal Masses

Tumors of the GI tract, pancreas, liver and biliary tree can be detected, evaluated for operability and even perfused with chemotherapeutic agents.

7

PANCREATICO-BILIARY TRACT EXAMINATIONS

A WIDE ASSORTMENT of diagnostic procedures are available for solving clinical problems involving the liver, bile ducts and pancreas. As was noted before, procedures with a high diagnostic sensitivity and accuracy are likely to be more difficult and expensive to perform and to involve greater discomforts and potential risks to the patient. Selection among these examinations must be made thoughtfully but promptly. Expeditious diagnosis may not make a big difference in the jaundiced victim of extensive pancreatic carcinoma, but you do not know that when you begin his workup. If he had, instead, a small stone impacted in his distal common bile duct, delays in discovering this could result in liver parenchymal damage, deterioration of clotting function, cholangitis and sepsis. These factors would greatly increase his risks for anesthesia and surgery.

The approach we shall take will be to consider five relatively distinct clinical presentations and to reason through the diagnostic considerations for each. The goal, of course, will be to reach a firm diagnosis permitting proper treatment, and to reach it in the shortest, safest, least expensive way.

Episodic Right Upper Quadrant Pain, Fatty Food Intolerance. R/O Gallstones

The AP plain film of the abdomen is a good starting point. After you take a systematic look at the entire image, you should direct particular attention to the right upper quadrant. About 20% of gallstones are calcified and are visible as round, faceted or ring-like opacities of variable number (Fig 7 – 1, A).

111

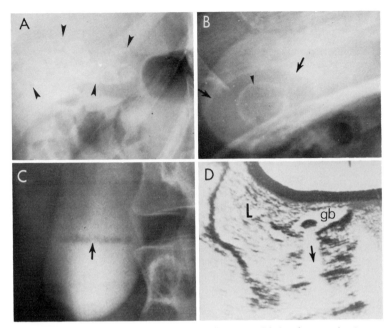

Fig 7–1.—Gallstones. **A,** plain film—multiple facetted stones *(arrowheads).* **B,** oral cholecystogram—single large stone *(arrows)* primarily lucent showing thin calcific inner shell *(arrowhead).* **C,** oral cholecystogram upright position; a thin layer of floating calculi *(arrow).* **D,** longitudinal ultrasound scan of right upper quadrant. Gallstone is causing acoustical shadow *(arrow).*

For most clinicians that radiographic finding, in this clinical setting, is good reason for cholecystectomy, unless other factors contraindicate it.

The oral cholecystogram has provided a sturdy diagnostic tool for many decades. Traditionally the patient is asked to ingest tablets of an organic iodine compound in the early evening and appear for abdominal filming the next morning. With luck, the patient brings a brightly opacified gallbladder, which is filmed in prone oblique, upright and decubitus positions. Stones appear as filling defects within the opacified bile (Fig 7–1 B, C). The process of opacification requires that the material dissolve, be absorbed, be taken up and conjugated by the liver and be excreted into the bile. The cystic duct

must be patent for the contrast material to enter the gallbladder.

Mechanisms which affect the solubility and intestinal
membrane transport of these compounds are complex and
result in unpredictable variations in absorption.[16] It is possible, therefore, to have a nonvisualizing gallbladder even in
the absence of gallbladder or liver disease. One quarter of
normal patients fail to show diagnostic opacification on the
first examination, but most of these will visualize the next
morning after a repeat dose. This has caused the patient the
inconvenience and anxiety of two visits to the x-ray department. A single visit regimen has been proposed[17] wherein the
patient takes tablets on 2 consecutive nights and comes in for
filming on the third morning. This greatly diminishes the
number of "repeat OCG" visits. Note that this is *not* a "double
dose" but a sequence of two single doses.

If, in a patient with good liver function, the gallbladder still
fails to visualize, the likelihood of its being diseased is high.
Obviously it remains to be determined whether noncalcified
stones are present in that nonvisualized gallbladder. A few
years ago, that was the informational stopping point, and management decisions were then made by weighing the radiologic odds and the clinical impression. We can give you a greater
degree of certainty now.

Cholecystosonography is the formal name for ultrasonic
examination of the gallbladder (GB ultrasound). In skilled
hands, 95% of gallbladders can be located and imaged.[18]
Stones reflect the beam back to the transducer, and areas behind them show "acoustical shadowing" (Fig 7–1, D). Accuracy of stone detection has been greatly improved recently by
the use of gravitational principles, as in radiography of the
gallbladder; these include upright and decubitus ultrasound
scans for layered or floating stones.

Acute RUQ Pain, Tenderness, Fever. R/O Acute Cholecystitis

If clinical and laboratory findings are absolutely typical, no
x-ray studies may be needed. Plain films and ultrasound scans

can be used to see if stones are present. Occasionally, the situation is not clear-cut; other entities such as pancreatitis, atypically located appendicitis or liver abscess are under consideration.

Intravenous cholangiography can help in this setting. This organic iodine compound is administered intravenously, is immediately taken up and excreted by hepatocytes and opacifies the extrahepatic bile ducts within minutes after administration. Filming, done every few minutes, is supplemented by tomography when maximal opacification has been achieved. If the cystic duct is patent, the gallbladder will also opacify after a variable delay. In patients with acute cholecystitis, the cystic duct is generally occluded by stone, debris or inflammatory edema. Therefore, visualization of the gallbladder is strong evidence against acute cholecystitis, and other explanations for the clinical problem must be sought.

Upper Abdominal Pain, Tenderness and ? Mass; Past Episodes of Vomiting, History of Alcoholism. R/O Pancreatic Disease, Gastric Neoplasm

After a plain film on which pancreatic calcifications are sought, an *upper GI series* would be performed to look for gastroduodenal neoplasm or ulcer, but also to check for varices along the way. The radiologist looks for intrinsic disease of the upper gut and for extrinsic displacement of the stomach and duodenum (Fig 7–2, A). If peristaltic activity is very active in the duodenum, interfering with assessment of its configuration, *hypotonic duodenography* with glucagon can be employed.

Ultrasound or *computed tomography* can provide imaging of the pancreas, showing masses or cysts (Fig 5–9, A). Ultrasound is less expensive, but if the patient is obese or has very substantial quantities of intestinal gas, computed tomography would be a better choice. CT, incidentally, does less well in very thin patients who lack the internal fat planes for density differential. Neither modality will do well unless you cleaned out the barium from the earlier upper GI series.

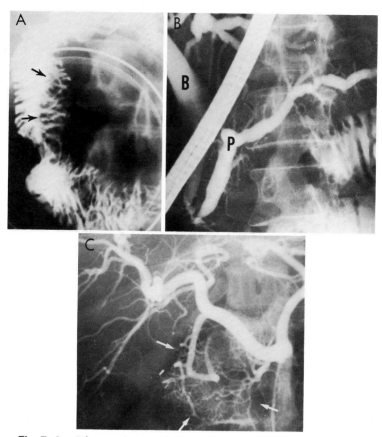

Fig 7–2.—Pancreatic abnormalities. **A,** duodenal loop showing medial indentation *(arrows)* by pancreatic mass. **B,** endoscopic retrograde cholangiography showing chronic pancreatitis with irregularly dilated pancreatic duct (P). Mild dilatation of bile duct (B) also present. **C,** celiac arteriogram showing hypervascular mass in pancreatic head.

If at this point diagnosis of a pancreatic pseudocyst is established, management considerations arise regarding surgery and its timing. *Angiography* is often carried out to exclude complications of pseudocyst such as splenic vein thrombosis or arterial erosion which has led to pseudoaneurysm.

If CT or ultrasound findings leave the pancreatic status uncertain, *endoscopic retrograde pancreatography* may provide definitive answers. In this sophisticated procedure, the endoscopist and radiologist collaborate to achieve opacification of the pancreatic duct system. A lateral-viewing fiberduodenoscope is passed; the ampulla of Vater is inspected and cannulated, and a fluoroscopically controlled contrast injection is made into pancreatic ducts (Fig 7-2, B). Fine detail of duct morphology is filmed in appropriate projections looking for obstructions, strictures, dilatations and displacements. Cytologic specimens are obtained, and, in addition, retrograde cholangiography may be performed. If a mass is found, angiography may help (Fig 7-2, C) to determine its extent and potential operability.

Jaundice and Itching. R/O Extrahepatic Biliary Obstruction

Before a radiologist is likely to see a requisition like this, a good deal of clinical and laboratory decision making had occurred. Clinical history and laboratory tests had indicated that a diagnosis of hepatocellular disease could reasonably be excluded. The question now centers on intrahepatic cholestasis versus mechanical obstruction of the major bile ducts. Commonest causes of the latter are pancreatic head carcinoma and choledocholithiasis; other causes are strictures or tumors of the common bile ducts. Figure 7-3 describes the algorithm (branching logic problem solving) in this situation. Both *ultrasound* and CT can provide good cross-sectional imaging of the liver to determine whether the intrahepatic ducts are dilated (Fig 7-4).

Although that decision might influence the choice of *endoscopic retrograde cholangiography (ERCP) or percutaneous transhepatic cholangiography (PTC)* to opacify the extrahepatic ducts (Fig 7-5), in many ways the two techniques are now interchangeable. With the new "skinny" (23 gauge) needle* technique for PTC, there are virtually no complications; nondilated intrahepatic ducts can be entered, and the cost is substantially less than that for ERCP. ERCP is suitable

---

*Developed in Chiba, Japan.

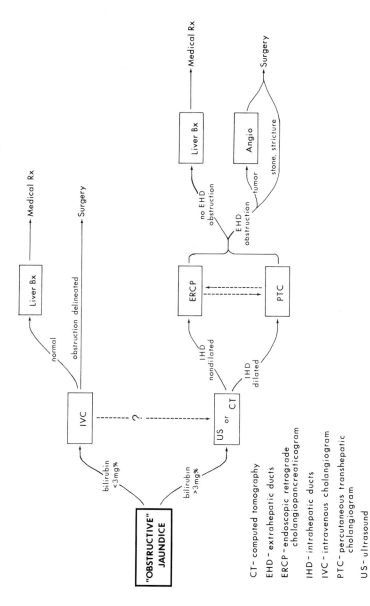

CT - computed tomography

EHD - extrahepatic ducts

ERCP - endoscopic retrograde
       cholangiopancreaticogram

IHD - intrahepatic ducts

IVC - intravenous cholangiogram

PTC - percutaneous transhepatic
      cholangiogram

US - ultrasound

Fig 7–3.—X-ray problem solving in jaundice.

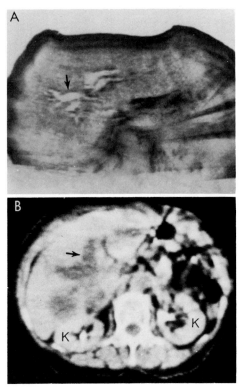

Fig 7-4. — Dilated intrahepatic bile ducts *(arrows)*. **A,** transverse sonography. **B,** computed tomography with contrast enhancement. K = kidney.

for both dilated and nondilated ducts and permits a more comprehensive approach, including pancreatography and cytologic studies at the ampulla. PTC requires adequate clotting function. Both studies are relatively new, and your hospital may not yet have a balance of skills and enthusiasm in both. Eventually, their relative roles and indications will solidify.[19] If the study performed shows extrahepatic biliary obstruction with a configuration suggesting neoplasm, *angiography* would be used for preoperative staging decisions.

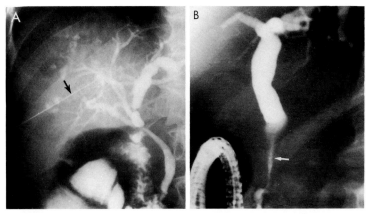

Fig 7–5.—Bile duct studies. **A,** percutaneous transhepatic cholangiography showing multiple strictures. Note needle *(arrow)*. **B,** endoscopic retrograde cholangiography showing stricture *(arrow)* and proximal dilatation.

R/O Common Duct Stones

Cholecystectomy Five Minutes Ago

During the course of cholecystectomy, the common duct is sometimes explored for stones. In addition to direct observation and instrumentation of the duct, x-ray opacification may be used. *Operative cholangiography* involves direct injection and filming of the extrahepatic ducts in the operating room with the patient anesthetized and the abdomen open. This is obviously not the time for substandard films, repeats and delays. The operating room portable x-ray machine must be effective; a radiographic technique must have been tried and corrected on an early scout film; ventilation must be suspended; the duct must be injected (without bubbles) at the right moment. Opportunities for fumbling abound, but the final result must be a film of good enough technical quality to show whether or not there are retained stones.

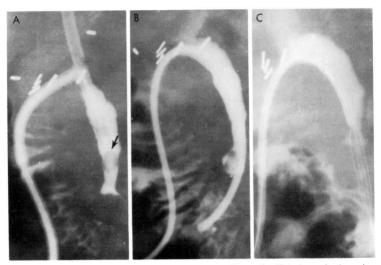

Fig 7–6.—Nonoperative stone extraction. **A,** T-tube cholangiogram discloses stone *(arrow)*. **B,** steerable catheter manipulated past stone. **C,** stone-basket engages stone, permitting extraction.

Cholecystectomy Ten Days Ago

At the close of a common duct exploration, a T-tube is left in the duct, with its long limb exiting laterally from the patient to provide postoperative drainage. At the end of 10 to 14 days the tube is ready for removal, but a last check for stones is made by means of a *T-tube cholangiogram.* Under fluoroscopic control, the tube is injected, and the ducts are searched for stones (Fig 7–6, A). If there are none, the tube is removed; normal biliary continuity will be established, and the fistula will close. If there are stones in the duct, that is a *big* problem. First of all, where did they come from? Were they missed on the operative cholangiogram? Did they drop from large intrahepatic branches? More importantly, however, what happens next? Until recently, a second operation was required. There is now another option which is safer and less expensive.

Cholecystectomy Five Weeks Ago

Nonoperative stone extraction.[20] When a retained stone is detected, the T-tube is left in place an additional 3 to 4 weeks to ensure a well-formed fistulous tract. After the T-tube is reinjected to ascertain that the stone is still there, the tube is removed. A special catheter with a steerable, controllable tip is advanced through the fistula and common bile duct to a point just beyond the stone (Fig 7–6, B). A tiny wire stonebasket is advanced through the catheter, is opened, engages the stone and is then withdrawn (Fig 7–6, C).

Cholecystectomy Two Years Ago

Consider the patient who did well after uncomplicated cholecystectomy 2 years ago but who has been having episodes of right upper quadrant pain and jaundice which subside spontaneously. The suspicion is that a stone is rattling around in the duct. Before it impacts and the patient becomes really sick, you want a definitive diagnosis. Assuming his bilirubin is reasonable (under 3 mg%), *intravenous cholangiography* might be performed to look for intraluminal filling defects. Alternatively, percutaneous transhepatic cholangiography could be employed. If a stone is found, the patient needs surgery.

8

URINARY TRACT RADIOLOGY

Perspective

BEFORE TRYING TO PREDICT the potential role of x-ray studies in your patient with urinary tract disease, you must keep in mind that many entities which produce profound functional derangement exhibit little gross morphologic disturbance. A whole gamut of "medical nephropathies" includes varieties of chronic glomerular, tubular and interstitial disease, as well as cortical and tubular necrosis.. For these individuals urography has nothing to offer, and the chemical and needle biopsy findings will determine their management.

In a large variety of other problems x-ray studies can provide you with important data for decision making. Among these problems are recurrent infection, stone formation, obstruction, suspected tumor, cystic disease and renovascular disease. Significant suspicion of one of these entities is a good indication for urography. Serious reactions to contrast agents can occur; it is necessary to weigh the potential risks and gains for your particular patient. The key question again should always be "what for?" not "why not?"

Preparation for Urography

The examination needs to be described and explained to the patient. He should be questioned about allergies and experiences with previous examinations. An occasional patient will equate the word "allergy" with pollens and pillows and neglect to tell you that he had to be resuscitated a few years ago when he had a "kidney test."

To prevent obscuration of renal detail by overlying feces,

123

cleansing of the colon is a necessity. This is often accomplished by a 1-day fluid diet followed by a strong cathartic on the evening before examination. In patients with normal renal function, part of the preparation should include fluid restriction, resulting in denser urographic opacification and better anatomic detail. If renal failure is present, however, dehydration must *not* be carried out because of the potential danger of protein precipitation in the renal tubules of oliguric proteinuric patients.

Study Method

Background

As you sort out and display the films later in the day, try to reconstruct the sequence of events that actually occurred that morning. The radiologist read your request form, concurred that the examination was indicated, requestioned the patient regarding allergies and had the technician proceed with a scout film. After studying it, the radiologist decided on the kind of urogram to be done, administered the contrast agent and then directed and evaluated the films as they were made. The findings on each film guided the selection of timing and projection for the next films.[38] The entire examination may have been completed in half an hour or prolonged over several hours in cases of obstruction or delayed function.

Viewing Technique

Scout

This is the preliminary AP film of the abdomen taken before the intravenous injection of contrast agent.

Evaluation of the Bowel Prep. — That the urogram was performed indicates that the radiologist was either satisfied with the preparation or cognizant that he was performing the urogram as an emergency procedure (i.e., no one schedules renal colic). Trying to "blast through" a loaded colon on a nonemergency renal workup is irresponsible and can doom the patient to a repeat examination unless tomography is available.

Study as an Abdominal Plain Film.—Note any abnormal findings with or without relation to the urinary tract. Do your "nonurinary" looking and deciding first; otherwise you may forget to do them later. Then search the area of the kidneys, ureters and bladder. This film may offer the last chance to see tiny opaque urinary calculi which would later be obscured by the contrast agent.

NEPHROGRAM PHASE

The tri-iodinated benzoic acid derivatives used for urography are excreted primarily by glomerular filtration.[21] On the earliest films, while contrast medium is still in the renal tu-

Fig 8–1.—Normal excretory urograms **A** and **B**. Note differences in morphology between the 2 patients.

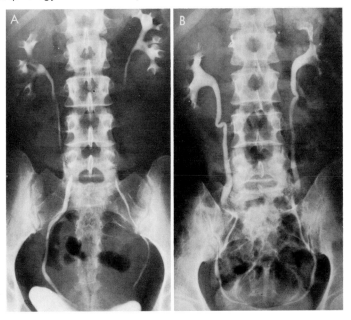

bules, the kidney parenchyma becomes diffusely opaque. This is an excellent opportunity to evaluate the size, shape and parenchymal homogeneity of the kidneys.

COLLECTING SYSTEM SEQUENCE

Over the next 20 minutes a sequence of films is obtained which delineates the conducting elements of the urinary tract (Fig 8 – 1).

Pelvis and Calices. — These are discussed in detail below.

Ureters. — In order to evaluate caliber and course, you must piece the images together because peristaltic activity results in visualization of random segments on any given film. Non-opaque ureteral calculi are invisible on the scout film but cause filling defects and consequent obstructive dilatation. Strategically placed retroperitoneal masses cause ureteral deviation.

Bladder. — (1) Filling defects: tumors, blood clots, nonopaque calculi, ureteroceles, Foley catheter balloons; (2) hypertrophic trabeculation; (3) extrinsic deformities — prostate, uterus, sigmoid colon.

Variations on a Urogram

Nephrotomography

At many hospitals tomographic cuts (traditional, not computed tomography) are a part of every standard urogram and in that sense should not be considered in the "variations" section. This is not universal, however, and the procedure is sometimes carried out only when x-ray or clinical findings raise questions concerning intrarenal masses or cysts.

Tomography during early vascular and nephrogram phases provides exceptionally sharp detail of the solid renal parenchyma and has far greater sensitivity for detecting small masses than the later phases of the urogram. Atrophic postinflammatory or postischemic scars are also very well-delineated.

Hypertensive Urography

In patients with suspected renovascular hypertension, a very early filming sequence after injection may be used to detect asymmetrically delayed function. Other clues include a small kidney which washes out poorly with forced diuresis and a ureter which is "notched" by large collateral arteries. The reliability and specificity of this study are not perfect, but it is a fairly good screening test when used in conjunction with other clinical parameters.

If screening studies suggest the possibility of remediable renal arterial disease, angiographic procedures are indicated. Renal vein catheterization and sampling for renin assay can be done, as well as renal arteriography to define the arterial abnormality.

High-Dose Urography

In urography of patients with moderate renal impairment (blood urea nitrogen [BUN] over 50; creatinine 2–4 mg%), the standard dose of contrast material is likely to yield poor visualization. High-dose urography, especially when augmented by tomography, can usually provide a nephrogram which is dense enough to show renal size and shape, plus later films which have enough pyelocaliceal detail to exclude obstructive uropathy.

Within the past few years, ultrasound, with increasing reliability, has begun providing similar information. As ultrasound is more widely and skillfully employed, the need for high-dose urography will diminish.

If neither ultrasound nor tomography confidently excludes obstruction, *retrograde pyelography* can be employed. This involves instrumentation in which cystoscopy is performed and the ureteral orifices are cannulated and injected with contrast material.

Urographic Interpretation

Anatomic Variants

Substantial variations in the configuration of the collecting systems exist and are related to the undisciplined branching habits of ureteric buds. These variants must, of course, be distinguished from renal disease. Building a broad baseline of normal variations involves looking at as many urograms as possible in life or in texts.[39]

Anomalies

Upper Tracts. — Horseshoe, crossed ectopia, congenital absence and pelvic locale are some of the more common renal anomalies. They are of more than theoretical significance because drainage may be impaired, predisposing to infection and stone formation.

Lower Tracts. — Anomalies of ureteral insertion, bladder development and urethral configurations constitute the common group of anomalies of this region. Most of these are not completely defined by excretory urography. In addition to clinical and cystoscopic examinations, *voiding cystourethrography* may be of assistance. The bladder is catheterized; contrast material is instilled, and the catheter is then removed. During voiding, films are taken to delineate the physiology and morphology. This study has its greatest application in the detection of obstructive urethral anomalies and vesico-ureteral reflux.

Diffuse Parenchymal Abnormalities

ENLARGED KIDNEYS

P olycystic disease
I nfiltration — amyloidosis, leukemia, lymphoma, glycogen storage disease
E dema — venous thrombosis, pyelonephritis, acute glomerulonephritis, acute obstruction

CONTRACTED KIDNEYS

    C hronic glomerulonephritis, chronic pyelonephritis
    H ypoplasia
    A trophy following obstruction
    I schemia — large vessel obstruction
    N ephrosclerosis — small vessel disease

Calcifications

Calculi. — Renal stones may vary from minute tubular concretions of medullary sponge kidney to huge "staghorn" calculi which form a cast of the entire pyelocaliceal system.

Nephrocalcinosis. — This is calcification deposited within the renal parenchyma. Dystrophic calcification occurs within damaged tissues, as is seen often in tuberculosis, occasionally in tumors and rarely in cysts. In tubular acidosis, and in hypercalcemic states such as hyperparathyroidism and sarcoidosis, diffuse calcification may develop in the medullary pyramids.

Focal Abnormalities

Scars. — In chronic pyelonephritis the medullary pyramid atrophies, the papillary tip withdraws from the calix, leaving it

Fig 8–2. — Sketch of chronic pyelonephritis with normal comparison. Note coarse, focal scarring and caliceal blunting.

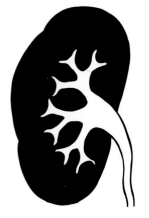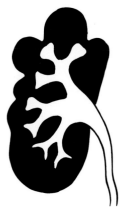

"clubbed," and the cortex becomes indented, The involvement is usually multifocal but often asymmetric (Fig 8–2). In tuberculosis there are similar findings but with increased tendency toward strictures, excavations and calcifications. Scars are not specific for inflammatory events; foci of segmental infarction can heal with similar configurations.

Filling Defects.—These are foci of radiolucency within any portion of the opacified collecting system. Differential considerations include nonopaque calculi, transitional cell neoplasm, blood clots, amorphous debris, sloughed papillae.

Masses.—An intrarenal, space-occupying lesion causes stretching and displacement of the collecting system. Differential

Fig 8–3.—X-ray workup of a renal mass.

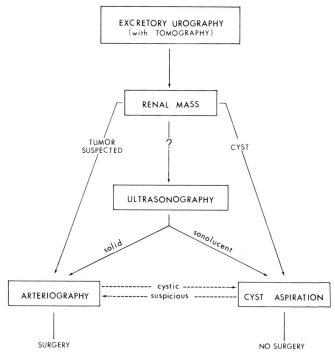

RENAL MASS WORKUP

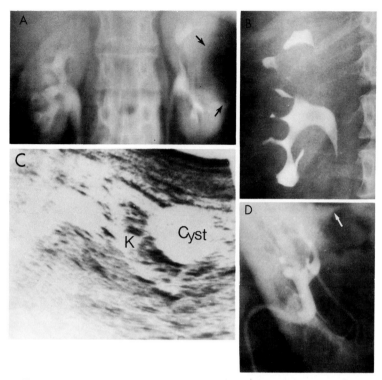

Fig 8–4.—Renal cystic lesions, multiple patients. **A,** nephrotomo-grams showing lucent lesion left kidney *(arrows).* **B,** excretory uro-gram in polycystic kidney. Note multifocal deformities. **C,** renal ultrasound showing sonolucent lesion tilting kidney. **D,** arteriogram of renal cyst. Note sharp beak *(arrow)* interface.

diagnosis includes: carcinoma, cyst, abscess, hematoma. If the spatial disturbances are multiple, polycystic disease is likely.

Figure 8–3 illustrates the radiologic approach to solution of the intrarenal mass problem, using another algorithm. Nephrotomography, ultrasonography and, more recently, computed tomography provide the first decision step regarding the probability of cystic versus solid lesion. Needle aspiration or arteriography is employed as the definitive maneuver.

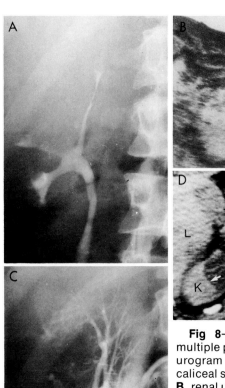

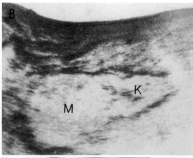

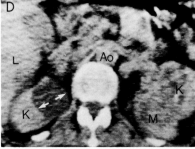

Fig 8–5.—Renal solid masses, multiple patients. **A,** excretory urogram showing upper pole caliceal stretching due to mass. **B,** renal ultrasound showing large mass (M) arising from upper pole. Multiple echoes in it indicate solid tissue. **C,** renal arteriogram showing malignant vasculature (less florid than Figure 4–1). **D,** computed tomography showing kidneys (K), high density mass (M) and low density cyst *(arrows)*. Ao-aorta, L-liver.

Figures 8–4 and 8–5 are a series of images showing the appearance of solid tumors and cysts with these various imaging modalities.

Ultrasound and CT in Nonneoplastic Problems

The new, noninvasive imaging modalities are delineating previously obscure pathologic conditions and, in some instances, providing an option for nonsurgical management.

- Following renal transplant surgery, ultrasound may be used to follow the renal size and shape (? rejection) and also to identify postoperative fluid collections related to leakage of urine or lymph.

- Serious abnormalities in the retroperitoneum such as perirenal abscess and perirenal hematoma can now be detected, localized for percutaneous drainage and followed by means of CT or ultrasound.

- When a kidney fails to visualize by excretory urography and no clearcut outlines are identified on plain films, ultrasound or CT can indicate whether congenital absence, chronic contraction or distal obstruction is responsible. The latter, of course, requires further delineation.

- When a distended, obstructed renal pelvis is identified, ultrasound or CT can guide percutaneous introduction of a small catheter into the renal pelvis. This can be used for antegrade pyelography defining the obstruction and can be exchanged for a larger catheter for use as a draining nephrostomy.[22]

9

RADIOLOGY OF THE FEMALE REPRODUCTIVE SYSTEM

FOR THE REASONS outlined in the section on radiation exposure, x-ray studies of the pelvis during the reproductive years should be kept to a minimum. Indications should be very clear-cut and the examinations performed in a way that assures maximum information with the least possible irradiation. These considerations obviously are of extreme importance during pregnancy and fade in significance when studies are needed for staging of a gynecologic malignancy.

Pregnancy

Ultrasonography is ideally suited for diagnostic work with the gravid uterus and has supplanted most of the traditional x-ray studies.[23] It was enthusiastically accepted because of its accuracy and the absence of radiation or other known potential hazards.

By 6 weeks after conception, the gestational sac is defined; by 8 weeks there are identifiable echoes from the fetus. Proper sequential increases in the cranial biparietal diameter provide assurance of healthy fetal growth when past history or clinical findings raise questions. Fetal abnormalities such as anencephaly, hydrocephaly and erythroblastosis are readily diagnosed, as is fetal demise. Polyhydramnios and hydatidiform mole also produce characteristic images (Fig 9 – 1).

The placenta is first imaged at about 10 weeks. Thereafter its location and configuration are readily documented, providing precise information concerning placenta previa or abruptio. Of historical interest only, now, is a body of information on

135

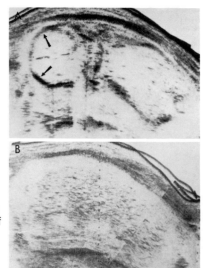

Fig 9–1. — Ultrasound of six-month pregnancies. **A,** normal fetus in breech presentation. Note normal head *(arrows).* **B,** hydatidiform mole showing diffusely granular pattern of echoes.

placenta previa as seen on plain films, radionuclide studies and angiography.

A lingering role for radiography continues to be *pelvimetry,* used on occasions when clinical pelvic examination or history of problems during previous labor raise questions concerning the adequate dimensions of the bony pelvis. Several methods are employed, but all have as their goal measurement of transverse and AP diameters at various pelvic levels. Measurements taken directly from the films are corrected for magnification, using films of a suitably positioned metal perforated ruler. The precision of these measurements is often offset by unmeasurable variations in pelvic soft tissues, the forces of labor and fetal cranial molding.

Infertility

When it is suspected that infertility is due to structural abnormality of the female reproductive system, two x-ray studies are often helpful:

Hysterosalpingography. — Under fluoroscopic control, sterile opaque contrast material is introduced into the uterus, outlining its cavity and the fallopian tubes. Congenital anomalies, adhesions and intraluminal masses can be identified. The patency of the tubes can be directly visualized by recording "spill" into the pelvic peritoneum.

Pelvic Pneumography (Gynecography). – A large volume of soluble, sterile gas is introduced into the peritoneal cavity by puncture through the anterior abdominal wall. With the patient in Trendelenburg position, gas rises into the pelvis, and films show the size, shape and location of the ovaries. Aplastic, hypoplastic and polycystic ovaries constitute the commonest positive findings. In the present state of technical development, sonography can delineate ovaries only if they are enlarged or cystic.

Miscellaneous Obstetric/Gynecologic Problems

The "Lost" IUD

An absent nylon thread on pelvic examination could have several explanations: The intrauterine device (IUD) has been expelled without the patient being aware of it. The thread has become detached or has retracted upward The IUD has perforated and is in an extrauterine location.

The simplest, least expensive first step would be a single AP film centered on the pelvis. The IUD is opaque; its presence or absence will be obvious. If it is present, further plain filming will not conclusively establish an intrauterine or extrauterine location. Before sonography, hysterosalpingography was the next step. The sonogram however, can show an echo pattern from the device and determine whether it is in the endometrial canal. We could start with sonography; however expulsion is so common that the cost of sonography for the initial screen is probably not justified

Postoperative Hematocrit Drop

After gynecologic (or any other) surgery, hematomas can be identified by ultrasound and their volume estimated. Followup examination can be used to show whether they are resolving or expanding and can guide the decision regarding need for surgical drainage.

Gynecologic Neoplasms

A number of very useful imaging techniques are available when detection and staging of pelvic neoplasm are necessary.

Ovarian Masses.—Plain films may show a soft tissue pelvic mass displacing normal bowel gas. Dermoids occasionally cooperate by displaying calcifications, teeth or fat.

Ultrasound can delineate the size and shape of the pelvic mass, display its solid or cystic characteristics and establish its extrauterine nature (Fig 9–2, A).

Carcinomas of the Uterine Cervix and Endometrium.—These

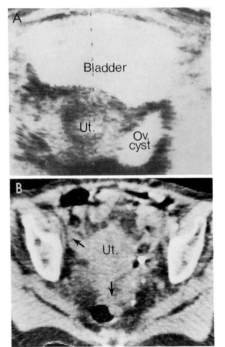

Fig 9–2.—Gynecologic imaging. **A,** transverse ultrasound scan through distended bladder, first trimester pregnancy (Ut), ovarian cyst. **B,** computed tomography of patient with carcinoma of the cervix, showing uterine mass (Ut) with extension posteriorly and laterally *(arrows).*

neoplasms are detected by pelvic examination, Pap smears and endometrial curettement; the radiologic contribution comes in their staging for proper management.

Urography and barium enema are often employed to exclude the possibility of spread of neoplasm to the bladder, ureters or rectum.

Computed tomography can show the overall bulk of the extrauterine extension, laterally along the parametria and anteroposteriorly toward other organs (Fig 9–2, B).

Lymphangiography is another technique used because the lymphatics are a major route of spread of these neoplasms, which eventually reach nodes of the common iliac and para-aortic group. These nodes can be opacified by infusion of an iodinated oil contrast medium into lymphatics on the dorsum of the feet. Identifying and cannulating those lymphatics involves injection of a blue dye intradermally, a short cutdown and a careful mini-dissection. Slow infusion of the contrast medium results in prompt opacification of lymphatic channels

Fig 9–3.—Lymphangiography. **A,** normal nodal size and architecture. **B,** carcinomatous filling defects *(arrow).* **C,** foamy nodes as in lymphoma.

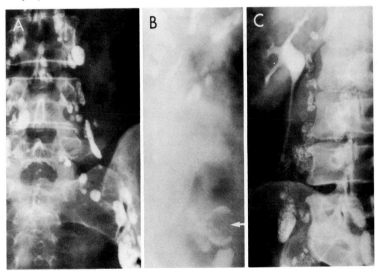

of the retroperitoneum and later nodal fill, filmed after 24 hours. Macroscopic carcinomatous implants in the nodes appear as focal filling defects (Fig 9-3). As you would expect from your pathology studies, lymphoma or marked hyperplasia results in a more diffusely enlarged, foamy pattern. (Lymphangiography is a major staging procedure in lymphoma patients.)

Once the nodes fill with the oil micro-droplets, they remain opacified for months, permitting plain abdominal films to be used to follow response to treatment.

Local anesthetic and a stack of magazines make this procedure relatively tolerable for the patient, but she must be able to maintain quiet supinity for about 2 hours. Pulmonary function must also be adequate because those infused oil droplets which are not taken up by the nodes travel via cisterna chyli and thoracic duct to the right heart and pulmonary capillaries. A poor diffusing capacity is a contraindication to lymphangiography.

Breast Disease

One out of every 14 of your female patients will develop breast cancer, and a much larger number will at some time have signs or symptoms of fibrocystic disease. Rational management of breast disease requires that you teach your patients breast self-examination and that you perform your physical examinations with care.

Mammography is extremely valuable in some settings and predictably useless in others. In most patients in their twenties and in many nulliparous women in their thirties, the normal fibroglandular breast parenchyma is very dense and obscures the soft tissue image of a growing carcinoma. Mammography, then, offers little in diagnosis or confident exclusion of cancer, and clinical parameters are the sole determinant of management.

With increasing age and parity, the breast background becomes more fatty, and diagnostic visibility begins. Tumors that are too small to be palpated may be visible as tiny spicu-

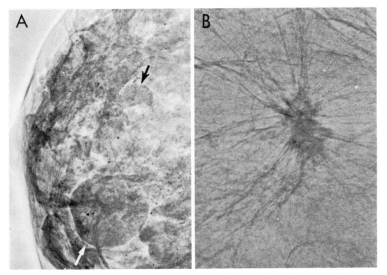

Fig 9–4.—Mammograms. **A,** gross fibrocystic disease showing diffuse calcification and multiple cysts *(arrows).* **B,** 1.5 cm malignant, spicculated lesion in clinically negative breast.

lated soft tissue foci, often at a stage when spread to the lymph nodes has not yet occurred (Fig 9–4).[24, 40] The coexistence of mammographic accuracy and breast cancer prevalence within the middle-aged and elderly group obviously is very fortunate. Additionally, in the older breast, epithelium seems less sensitive to potential radiation oncogenesis effects. Concerns about exposure, therefore, should be far overshadowed by risks of missing an early, curable lesion.

10

SKULL FILMS AND NEURORADIOLOGIC PROCEDURES

Perspectives

NEURORADIOLOGY is an enormous field with excellent author-itative texts[41, 42] and a rapidly expanding literature of tech-niques and applications. For the radiologist, neurologist and neurosurgeon, the challenges and satisfactions of pinpoint accuracy and aggressive therapeutics are present in abun-dance. This is an area, however, in which younger clinicians often seem intimidated. The intern who so obviously enjoys discussing his patient's chest, abdomen and bone films with the radiologist becomes visibly discouraged, apathetic or hos-tile when the skull films are presented. Systematic analysis of a skull examination should permit you to extract and under-stand the significant findings. You should also know enough about the special procedures to discuss them intelligently with your consultants.

Skull films are a notoriously overrequested examination, with the result that their overall yield is poor. When the intern who "never finds anything" on skull x-rays reviews his recent rather frequent requests, he will find trivial trauma, "spells," diabetic coma, uremic encephalopathy, heart block, drug over-dose and hypoglycemic attacks heading the list, all in patients with no localizing neurologic findings. In those settings waste of effort and money was predictable. There was, in addition, an element of potential hazard in transporting and positioning obtunded patients with intubated airways, IVs, pacemakers

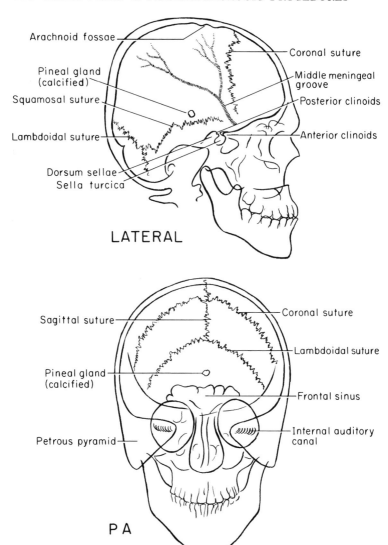

Fig 10–1. – Normal skull sketches, lateral and PA.

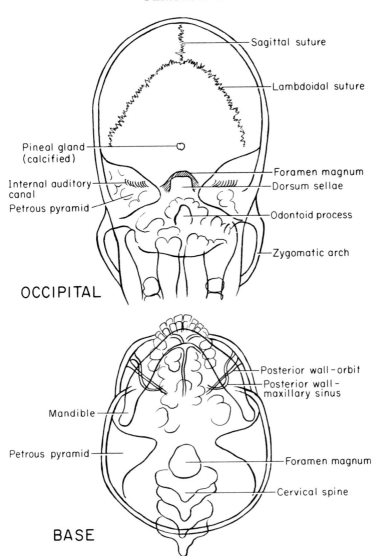

Fig 10–2. — Normal skull sketches, occipital and base views.

and monitoring leads. To anticipate your next suggestion, portable skull films are almost as good as portable abdominal films.

Skull Films: Study Method

Orientation

The basic projections are the PA, lateral, occipital (Towne) and base view (Figs 10–1 and 10–2). Utilizing an anatomy book and innate cunning, visualize how these were taken.
Note: In the setting of trauma, one of the lateral films is often made with a horizontal beam to detect air-fluid (blood) levels in the sinuses. Standard skull films are often made with a vertical beam, which cannot ever show an air-fluid level.

The Cranium

Search the bone for lucent or sclerotic foci, fractures, widened or prematurely fused sutures.

NORMAL RADIOLUCENCIES

Sutures are in characteristic locations and show finely interdigitated surfaces.

Vascular markings are semilucent grooves, also in dependable locations. Identify those for the meningeal arteries, dural venous sinuses, parasagittal fossae for the arachnoid granulations, randomly scattered small venous channels and diploic lakes.

FRACTURES

A *linear fracture* is straight, sharply delineated, nonbranching and intensely radiolucent.

A *depressed fracture* is obvious only if the beam hits the defect and fragment in perfect profile (Fig 10–3, A). (With a spherical object like a skull, that will often *not* be the case.) Look carefully for an area of *increased opacity* where the density of the depressed fragment overlaps that of the intact skull.

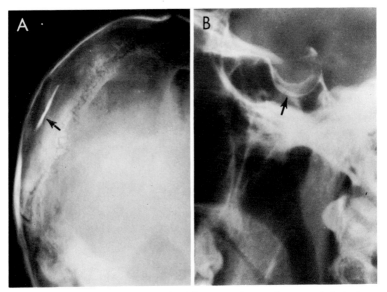

Fig 10-3.—A, depressed skull fracture *(arrow)* on occipital view. **B**, asymmetrically enlarged sella turcica *(arrow)* on lateral view.

Basilar fractures are sometimes impossible to detect on plain films. Indirect clues should be sought, such as fluid levels in a sinus or clouding of temporal bone air cells by blood.

Sella Turcica

This structure is easily seen on standard lateral projection and should be evaluated for size, shape and mineralization. Abnormality can take the form of generalized expansion, focal bone destruction or pathologic calcification. Pituitary adenomas and craniopharyngiomas are the commonest lesions to affect the sella turcica; however chordomas, aneurysms and optic gliomas are not rare (Fig 10-3, B).

Pineal Calcification

The pineal is normally in the midline. If visibly calcified, it can tell us of important intracranial shifts.

Whose pineal is calcified? You can assume that children and adolescents will not have pineal calcification. The incidence increases with age, approximating 20% in patients in their twenties and 70% in patients in their seventies.

What film shows it best? If you cannot confidently point to it on the lateral film where the overlying calvarium is flat and simple, do not trust what you *think* you see on PA projection. It would be a serious error to misinterpret overlapping calvarial bone densities as pineal gland and draw conclusions about intracranial shifts.

What if the PA film is slightly rotated? While no one sanctions bad films, it is a fact of life that optimum positioning is difficult in obtunded or combative patients. Fortunately, because of its location near the coronal plane of the odontoid, the pineal rotates relatively little on PA films where the frontal and occipital bones are hopelessly misaligned. Judgment of its position relative to the midline remains valid.

A Search for Other Intracranial Calcifications

Normal.—Choroid plexuses of the lateral ventricles, falx or tentorial dural plaques.

Abnormal and Distinctive.—Carotid atherosclerosis, basilar artery aneurysm, meningeal vascular malformation (Sturge-Weber), granulomas, basal ganglia calcifications, toxoplasmosis, cytomegalic inclusion disease, tuberous sclerosis.

Abnormal but Noncharacteristic.—Tumors (meningeal and gliomatous), old infarcts, some infections.

Significance of Skull Fractures

The neurologic status of the patient and the possibility of intracranial hemorrhage are the real considerations in managing head trauma victims. The presence or absence of an associated skull fracture usually does not influence management.[25] There are three exceptions to this:

- A fracture which crosses the middle meningeal groove alerts you to the possibility of arterial bleeding and an epidural hematoma.

- A fracture which enters a mastoid or paranasal sinus communicates with a potentially contaminated space. You may wish to use antibiotics (controversial).
- A depressed fracture may cause injury to underlying brain cortex and lead to an epileptogenic focus. Most neurosurgeons would remove or elevate the fragment.

Signs of Increased Intracranial Pressure

In children, reliable signs include widened sutures and erosion of portions of the sella turcica. The finding of prominent

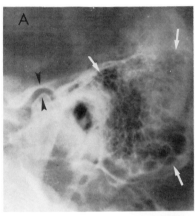

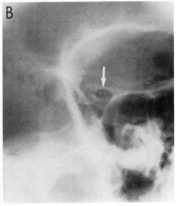

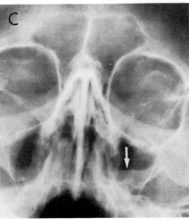

Fig 10–4.—Modified projections for craniofacial problems. **A,** mastoid region in angulated lateral view. Pneumatized area of temporal bone *(arrows).* Temporomandibular joint *(arrowheads).* **B,** optic foramen *(arrow)* showing on oblique projection through orbit. **C,** Water's view shows orbits, facial bones and sinuses. Note air-fluid level *(arrow)* in left maxillary antrum.

"convolutional" markings on the inner surface of the skull is often cited, but because this can be seen in some normals, it is not diagnostic as an isolated finding.

In adults, effects are primarily demineralization and erosion of the posterior portion of the sella turcica.

Papilledema is generally present before plain film signs of increased pressure develop.

Modifications for Special Problems

Although the standard skull examination is a good survey of craniofacial structures, certain problems require modified projections and positions for their solution (Fig 10–4). Examples of such areas include:

mastoids
sinuses
orbits
facial bones
optic foramina

Special Techniques in Neuroradiology

Radionuclide Brain Scans

Certain intravenously administered radioactive materials localize in intracranial foci where there has been an alteration in the blood-brain barrier. Positive scans may be seen in a variety of circumstances: neoplasms, hematomas, infarcts, abscesses and even certain demyelinating diseases (Fig 10–5).

A sophisticated modification is *radionuclide angiography*, the rapid recording of images of an isotope bolus after intravenous injection. This can provide a rough outline of intracranial arterial flow and identify certain vascular lesions and occlusions.

Radionuclide cisternography is a method of evaluating cerebrospinal fluid circulation in patients with nonobstructive hydrocephalus. Radioactive iodine labeled serum albumen is put into the lumbar subarachnoid space, and its distribution within the head is studied.

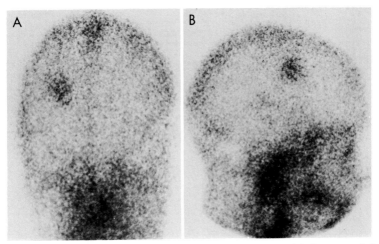

Fig 10–5.—Radionuclide brain scan in patient with intracranial metastasis. **A,** anterior. **B,** lateral scan.

Computed Tomography

The basic principles were described in Chapter 4, where it was pointed out that intracranial applications of CT have become well established and have caused substantial alterations in the traditional workup and management of central nervous system disease. Figure 10–6 shows a spectrum of lesions which are readily apparent on transverse axial imaging. Abnormalities of the ventricular system, the brain substance and the subdural space are sharply depicted. Although less expensive radionuclide scans show "hot spots" at brain tumors, they do not provide information regarding midline shift, ventricular distortion, surrounding edema or smaller, associated lesions.

CT scans are now showing that head trauma victims with subdural hematomas sometimes have associated brain contusions, accounting for their delayed recovery after appropriate subdural drainage.[26] Followup CT scans can show the adequacy of drainage and any reaccumulation of hematoma and can document the persistence or resolution of the cerebral contusions.

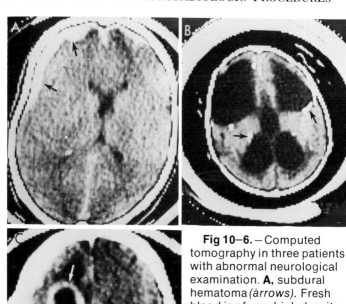

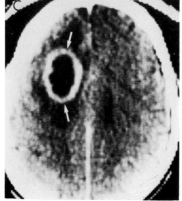

Fig 10–6. — Computed tomography in three patients with abnormal neurological examination. **A,** subdural hematoma *(arrows).* Fresh blood is of very high density. Note shift of normal-sized ventricular system. **B,** hydrocephalus and intracranial calcification *(arrows)* in young child with toxoplasmosis. **C,** brain tumor showing high density rim *(arrows)* after contrast material given intravenously for enhancement. Note surrounding edema of low density.

For certain clinical settings, a negative CT scan is adequate evidence concerning intracranial pathology, and the work-up can be terminated at that point. In some instances, for instance subdural hematomas, the CT scans are accepted as sufficient data, and surgical management can be instituted. Most neurosurgeons, however, would want angiographic information before attacking a brain tumor that was discovered on CT scan.

Arteriography

Intracranial arteriography is generally achieved by a transfemoral catheter approach via the aorta to the carotid and vertebral vessels. Occasionally direct puncture of the carotid artery in the neck is still performed. Biplane serial filming provides the full sequence of arterial, capillary and venous circulation for maximum morphologic and physiologic information. Geometric magnification and photographic subtraction

Fig 10–7.—Cranial arteriography in 4 patients. **A,** extracranial vascular disease. Large, posterior atherosclerotic plaque *(arrow)* at carotid bifurcation. **B,** berry aneurysm *(arrow)* at anterior communicating artery. **C,** arteriovenous malformation. **D,** subdural hematoma *(arrows)* displacing middle cerebral convexity branches and causing midline shift.

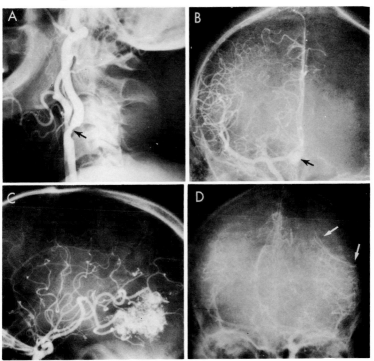

techniques are employed to study fine detail. Most would regard arteriography as the definitive procedure in tumors, arteriovenous malformations, aneurysms, hematomas and occlusive vascular disease (Fig 10 – 7).

Meticulously controlled selective embolization can be carried out with excellent results. Improvement is possible in patients with extensive, inoperable vascular malformations. Highly vascular brain tumors can be embolized preoperatively, permitting a faster, safer resection.

Air Encephalography

Pneumoencephalogram. — A small volume of gas is introduced into the subarachnoid space via lumbar puncture. With the patient seated in the upright position, the gas ascends to the head, whereupon a series of enlightened manipulations results in filling of the subarachnoid cisterns and ventricular cavities. Lesions within and adjacent to the ventricles and cisterns can be delineated.

Ventriculogram. — In this study gas is injected directly into the lateral ventricles via calvarial drill holes. This provides information about the ventricles but not about the cisternal spaces.

In the past these were the definitive procedures in deep intracranial masses, hydrocephaly, cerebral atrophy and degenerative central nervous system disease. As the capabilities of CT increase, the indications for air studies are diminishing.

Myelography

Iodinated contrast agent injected into the lumbar subarachnoid space is manipulated in a cephalad direction by controlled tilting of the fluoroscopic table. Specific configurations and deformities identify lesions as:

    extradural — herniated disc, metastatic tumor to spine
    intradural — meningioma, neurofibroma
    intramedullary — glioma, syrinx

Oil-based contrast agents are gradually being supplanted by water-soluble materials which provide better structural detail.

EPILOGUE

If you haven't noted the brevity and incompleteness of the contents of this manual, you haven't been paying attention. This was premeditated, and the manual was offered in this form without apology. Facts were often presented without discussion or defense in the expectation that as time and curiosity permitted, you would seek out supplementary information.

Material in this manual has been freely extracted from a variety of sources with only sketchy reference designation. This was done with confidence that those particular authors and educators would enthusiastically approve of any means that provided useful dissemination of their findings.

Answer Sheet

Figure 3–2
- **A** Scaphoid fracture.
- **B** Greenstick fracture radius; subtle nondisplaced bending fracture of ulna. A pneumatic splint is present.
- **C** Salter II epiphyseal fracture distal radius; nondisplaced, buckled fracture distal ulna.
- **D** Angulated ulna fracture with anteriorly dislocated proximal radius (Monteggia fracture).
- **E** Pathologic fracture.
- **F** Angulated fracture of surgical neck of humerus seen on transthoracic lateral view.

Figure 3–3
- **A** Healing "march" fracture third metatarsal neck.
- **B** Bi-malleolar ankle fracture with lateral displacement.
- **C** Subtle fracture of medial tibial plateau, required oblique view to capture fracture line in profile. Note cortical discontinuity just medial to tibial spines.
- **D** Femoral neck fracture with impaction.

Figure 3–4

   A Osteogenic sarcoma with invasion into adjacent soft tissues.

   B Benign, expansile, sharply corticated lesion (primarily fibrous) with pathologic fracture.

   C Osteomyelitis showing diffuse, permeative destruction with stripe of periosteal new bone formation.

Figure 3–9

   A Ischemic necrosis of femoral head. Note fragmentation and collapse of head while cartilage is preserved and acetabulum is normal.

   B Degenerative arthritis of knee; narrowing, sclerosis and osteophytes predominate medially.

   C Rheumatoid arthritis; narrowing and erosions at second and third MCP joints; swelling and erosion at second and fourth PIP joints.

   D Gout showing gross destruction of first metatarsophalangeal joints, smaller erosions proximally.

Figure 3–11

   A Multilevel degenerative arthritis showing narrowed discs, sclerosis and osteophytes.

   B C5-6 dislocation causing quadriparesis. This was a flexion injury in which C5 dislocated anteriorly. The facets are now "locked" with the inferior tip of the C5 facets *anterior* to the superior tips of the C6 facets. This level could not be seen on initial cross-table views until traction on his arms lowered his shoulders.

   C Bacterial spine infection showing irregularly narrowed disc, destroyed vertebral end-plates, reactive sclerosis and paraspinal swelling (review Fig 2–3).

   D Absent right transverse process L2. Past history of right nephrectomy for renal carcinoma. Tumor recurrence was invading adjacent spine.

   E One year later, destruction has progressed to involve pedicle, articulating facets and lamina.

SUGGESTED READING

Basic General Texts

1. Squire, L.: *Fundamentals of Radiology* (rev. ed.; Philadelphia: W. B. Saunders Co., 1975).
2. Meschan, I.: *Roentgen Signs in Clinical Practice*, Vols. I and II (Philadelphia: W. B. Saunders Co., 1966).
3. Sutton, D.: *Textbook of Radiology* (Edinburgh, Scotland: Churchill Livingstone, 1975).
4. Paul, L., and Juhl, I.: *Essentials of Roentgen Interpretation* (3d ed.; New York: Paul B. Hoeber, 1972).

Supplementary Articles

5. Antoku, S., and Russell, W.: Dose to active bone marrow, gonads and skin from roentgenography and fluoroscopy, Radiology 101:669, 1971.
6. Thomas, E. L.: Search behavior, Radiol. Clin. North Am. 7:403, 1969.
7. Figley, M.: Mediastinal minutiae, Semin. Roentgenol. 4: 22, 1969.
8. Steiner, R.: Radiology of pulmonary circulation, Am. J. Roentgenol. 91:249, 1964.
9. Heitzman, E. R., Ziter, F. M., et al.: Kerley's interlobular septal lines: Roentgen pathologic correlation, Am. J. Roentgenol. 100:578, 1967.
10. Fraser, R. G.: The radiologist and obstructive airway disease, Am. J. Roentgenol. 120:737, 1974.
11. Martel, W.: The patterns of rheumatoid arthritis in the hand and wrist, Radiol. Clin. North Am. 2:221, 1964.
12. Buddemeyer, E. U.: The physics of diagnostic ultrasound, Radiol. Clin. North Am. 13:391, 1975.
13. Evens, R. G., and Jost, R. G.: Economic analysis of computed tomography units, Am. J. Roentgenol. 127:191, 1976.
14. Cloe, L. E.: Health planning for computed tomography:

Perspectives and problems, Am. J. Roentgenol. 127:187, 1976.

15. Miller, R., and Nelson, S.: Roentgenologic demonstration of tiny amounts of free intraperitoneal gas, Am. J. Roentgenol. 112:574, 1971.

16. Berk, R. N., and Loeb, P. M.: Pharmacology and physiology of the biliary radiographic contrast materials, Semin. Roentgenol. 11:147, 1976.

17. Burhenne, H. J., and Obata, W. G.: Single visit oral cholecystography, N. Engl. J. Med. 292:627, 1975.

18. Leopold, G. R., Amberg, J., Gosink, B., and Mittelstaedt, C.: Gray scale ultrasonic cholecystography: A comparison with conventional radiographic techniques, Radiology 121:445, 1976.

19. Elias, E., Hamlyn, A. N., Jain, S., Long, R. G., Summerfield, J. A., Dick, R., and Sherlock, S.: A randomized trial of percutaneous transhepatic cholangiography versus endoscopic retrograde cholangiography for bile duct visualization in obstructive jaundice, Gastroenterology 71: 439, 1976.

20. Burhenne, H. J.: Non-operative retained biliary stone extraction, Am. J. Roentgenol. 117:388, 1973.

21. Talner, L. B.: Urographic contrast media in uremia: Physiology and pharmacology, Radiol. Clin. North Am. 10: 421, 1972.

22. Harris, R. D., McCullough, D. L., and Talner, L. B.: Percutaneous nephrostomy, J. Urol. 115:628, 1976.

23. Sanders, R. C., and Conrad, M. R.: Sonography in obstetrics, Radiol. Clin. North Am. 13:435, 1975.

24. Ferg, S. A., Shaber, G. S., Patchefsky, A., Schwartz, G. F., Edeiken, J., Libshitz, H. I., Nerlinger, R., Curley, R. F., and Wallace, J. D.: Analysis of clinically occult and mammographically occult breast tumors, Am. J. Roentgenol. 128:403, 1977.

25. Bell, R. S., and Loop, J. W.: The utility and futility of radiographic skull examination for injury, N. Engl. J. Med. 284:236, 1971.

26. Dublin, A. B., French, B. N., and Rennick, J. M.: Computed tomography in head trauma, Radiology 122:365, 1977.

Radiologic Hi-Fi Shelf

27. Felson, B.: *Fundamentals of Chest Roentgenology* (Philadelphia: W. B. Saunders Co., 1960).
28. Fraser, R. G. and Pare, J. P.: *Diagnosis of Diseases of the Chest* (Philadelphia: W. B. Saunders Co., 1970).
29. Heitzman, E. R.: *The Lung: Radiologic Pathologic Correlations* (St. Louis: C. V. Mosby Co., 1973).
30. Dahlgreen, S., and Nordenstrom, B.: *Transthoracic Needle Biopsy* (Chicago: Year Book Medical Publishers, Inc., 1966).
31. Murray, R., and Jacobson, H.: *The Radiology of Skeletal Disorders* (Baltimore: Williams & Wilkins Co., 1971).
32. Jaffe, H. L.: *Tumors and Tumorous Conditions of the Bones and Joints* (Philadelphia: Lea & Febiger, 1958).
33. Forrester, D. M., and Nesson, J. W.: *The Radiology of Joint Disease* (Philadelphia: W. B. Saunders Co., 1973).
34. Abrams, H.: *Angiography* (2d ed; Boston: Little, Brown and Co., 1971).
35. Carter, B. L., Morehead, J., Wolpert, S., Hammerschlag, S., Griffiths, H., and Kahn, P.: *Cross-sectional Anatomy. Computed Tomography and Ultrasound Correlation* (New York: Appleton-Century-Crofts, 1977).
36. Frimann-Dahl, J.: *Roentgen Examinations in Acute Abdominal Disease* (2d ed.; Springfield, Ill.: Charles C Thomas, Publisher, 1960).
37. Margulis, A. R., and Burhenne, H. J. (eds.): *Alimentary Tract Roentgenology* (St. Louis: C. V. Mosby Co., 1967).
38. Lalli, A.: *The Tailored Urogram* (Chicago: Year Book Medical Publishers, Inc., 1973).
39. Emmett, J. L., and Witten, D. M.: *Clinical Urography* (Philadelphia: W. B. Saunders Co. 1971).
40. Wolfe, J. N.: *Xeroradiography of the Breast* (Springfield, Ill.: Charles C Thomas, Publisher, 1972).
41. Taveras, J.: *Diagnostic Neuroradiology* (Baltimore: Williams & Wilkins Co., 1964).
42. Newton, T. H., and Potts, D. G.: *Radiology of the Skull and Brain* (St. Louis: C. V. Mosby Co., 1974).

43. Caffey, J.: *Pediatric X-Ray Diagnosis* (7th ed.; Chicago: Year Book Medical Publishers, Inc., 1978).
44. Simonton, J. H., and Jamison, R. C.: *An Outline of Radiographic Findings in Multiple-System Disease* (Springfield, Ill.: Charles C Thomas, Publisher, 1966).

INDEX

161